I have searched for a book like this for almost 13 years. This absolutely grabbed and kept my attention. I am just blown away, as I have prayed for such a tool to speak to my son in a loving way so he can see Christ working in him—even with T1D.
- Jill, parent of a child with diabetes

I've never really related scripture directly to my diabetes, but WOW! It all really does fit together! Publishing these kinds of stories not only continues to raise much needed awareness for diabetes, but also shouts the blessed news that God is good even to those of us living with a chronic illness.
- Sue, lives with type 1 diabetes

The topics you write about are very real and pertinent to any family dealing with diabetes. You easily relate the everyday hassles we deal with to the life of Jesus and the things that we know to be true about Him.
- Janna, parent of child with diabetes

These devotions are excellent, and something that I think is needed. I was disappointed when it ended.
- Dawn, lives with type 1 diabetes and parents a child with diabetes

Although I have type 2 diabetes and my issues and struggles can be different than yours with type 1, your devotions are relevant to the issues of dealing with any disease. You have a gift for writing and making this all so meaningful. It is relevant for many.
- Bev, lives with type 2 diabetes

This is a much-needed resource for all who are impacted by diabetes. There is such a small amount of encouraging, faith-based literature on this topic, and I am thrilled that you answered God's call to share your story.
- Laura, parent of a child with diabetes

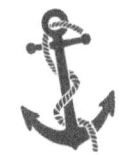

DEVOTIONS ON DIABETES:
A 30-Day Journey to Anchor Your Soul

KAYCEE PARKER

Devotions on Diabetes: A 30-Day Journey to Anchor Your Soul
©2023 Kaycee Parker, KP Communications

www.devotionsondiabetes.com

All rights reserved. This book contains material protected under International and Federal Copyright Laws and Treaties. Any unauthorized reprint or use of this material is prohibited. No part of this book may be reproduced, stored in a retrieval system, or transmitted in any form or by any means—electronic or mechanical, photocopying, recording, scanning, or other—without prior written permission from the author.

Scripture quotations marked (NIV) are taken from the Holy Bible, New International Version®, NIV®. Copyright ©1973, 1978, 1984, 2011 by Biblica, Inc.™ Used by permission of Zondervan. All rights reserved worldwide. www.zondervan.com. The "NIV" and "New International Version" are trademarks registered in the United States Patent and Trademark Office by Biblica, Inc.™

Scripture quotations marked (ESV) are from The ESV® Bible (The Holy Bible, English Standard Version®), copyright © 2001 by Crossway, a publishing ministry of Good News Publishers. Used by permission. All rights reserved.

Scripture quotations marked (NLT) are taken from the Holy Bible, New Living Translation, copyright ©1996, 2004, 2015 by Tyndale House Foundation. Used by permission of Tyndale House Publishers, Carol Stream, Illinois 60188. All rights reserved.

Any emphasis in scripture quotations have been added by the author.

Cover design: Annette Zacho
Back cover headshot: Courtney Smith Photography

Interior photography by: Sean Oulashin (page 25), Artem Kovalev (page 37), Ameen Fahmy (page 45), Samantha Lynch (page 57), Joe Pohle (page 69), Alessio Lin (page 81), Aleksandr Eremin (page 93), C Boyd (page 101), Khatam Tadayon (page 113), Jeff Hardi (page 121), and Clay Banks (page 129).

I am not a doctor. Content in this book is not medical advice.

ISBN: 978-0-9991973-2-5 (paperback)

*To all those fighting the fight,
you are not alone.*

Deuteronomy 31:8

CONTENTS

DAY 1: You Are Seen — 14

DAY 2: Charting Expectations — 18

DAY 3: Nothing Makes Sense — 22

DAY 4: The Wait — 26

DAY 5: Wandering Away — 30

DAY 6: Isolation — 34

DAY 7: Broken Design — 38

DAY 8: Unanswered Questions — 42

DAY 9: A Thankful Heart — 46

DAY 10: Permission to Mourn — 50

DAY 11: The Best Medicine — 54

DAY 12: The Carbs in Humble Pie — 58

DAY 13: A Call to Prayer — 62

DAY 14: Identity — 66

DAY 15: Embrace the Mystery — 70

DAY 16: Vacation Daydreams	74
DAY 17: Battle Weary	78
DAY 18: Sheer Magnitude	82
DAY 19: Becoming Interruptible	86
DAY 20: The Illusion of Control	90
DAY 21: True Value	94
DAY 22: Our Need for Dependence	98
DAY 23: A New Prayer	102
DAY 24: Generous Grace	106
DAY 25: From Fear to Prayer	110
DAY 26: Compression	114
DAY 27: Building Trust	118
DAY 28: Perfect Peace	122
DAY 29: Diabetes is Temporary	126
DAY 30: Drop Anchor	130

INTRODUCTION

May 5, 2022, marked thirty years of living with type 1 diabetes.

I had finished an online Bible reading plan with my husband and his sister earlier that year. We had journeyed through the gospel of John together, and part of one reading changed my perspective on diabetes forever.

> As he went along, he saw a man blind from birth. His disciples asked him, "Rabbi, who sinned, this man or his parents, that he was born blind?"
>
> "Neither this man nor his parents sinned," said Jesus, "but this happened so that the works of God might be displayed in him."
> John 9:1-3 (NIV)

After reading each day's chapter, we would post our thoughts in a group chat. This was my response that day:

> I have always wondered why I have diabetes that I manage every hour of every day. No one else in my family has type 1, I didn't do anything to bring it on, and doctors have told me they don't really know either. But we live in a world full of sickness and disease. And perhaps God allowed it because He wants me to glorify Him through it like He did with the blind man in John 9.
>
> When I am running high and feel like I have the flu, God is still good. When I can't yet eat because my number is high, God is still good. When I'm low and drinking a juice box like I'm a four-year-old kid, God is still good. When I'm counting carbs for my insulin dose, God is still good.

> Maybe His plan is to use it to shape and mold me to bring Him glory. Our struggles are not for nothing. He can use anything He wants!

This shifted my view of diabetes entirely. Previously, I was focused on dealing with highs and lows, and managing my disease as best I could (which, of course, I still do). But this new perspective has me thinking of ways I can point people to Jesus through it all. How can I use the talents and gifts God has given me, along with the challenges of this disease, to point people to Him and give Him glory? Perhaps one way I can give glory to God is by sharing with you through this devotional.

I do feel that I need to let you know that, although I am a pastor's wife, I'm not a pastor myself. I'm just a storyteller by nature who loves Jesus and lives with diabetes. I'm simply trying to take my experience with type 1, view it through the lens of the Bible, apply what I learn to my life, and share it with you.

My hope is not only will this glorify God, but it will also help you stay connected to the truth. This disease is a challenge, but being connected to the source of life is what gets us through. In all the storms we face, we are firm and secure when we are anchored in Him. So I want to encourage you to do a couple things as you make your way through this book.

1. Read God's Word every day.
That's why you will find additional readings listed within these devotions. God's Word is living and active, the writer of Hebrews tells us, and I pray He reaches you through His Word as you read the pages of this book and the additional readings suggested.

2. Think and pray.
Consider the questions and prayer prompts throughout this book as you go about your day.

May He use all these things to work in you and allow you a glimpse of His never-ending goodness through it all.

Can I pray for us as we get started together?

Lord, what a privilege it is to speak to people dealing with diabetes and point them to You in the midst of what we face. I thank You for putting this book on my heart and being with me in writing it. I pray that through this book You would reach those reading it in ways that only You can. Renew their minds. Draw them nearer to You. Show them Your love in tangible ways. Comfort them and protect them. Refresh their perspective. And encourage them to be anchored in You—our one true hope. Amen.

> WE HAVE THIS HOPE AS AN **ANCHOR FOR THE SOUL,** FIRM AND SECURE.
>
> Hebrews 6:19a (NIV)

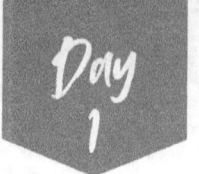

Day 1

YOU ARE SEEN

———

May 5, 1992. I remember it like it was yesterday.

My mother noticed the symptoms early on. The overnight trips to the bathroom. The tired, unmotivated *(and grumpy)* attitude. The unquenchable thirst. The weight loss. She had a suspicion it was type 1 diabetes because she knew a child who had recently been diagnosed after having these symptoms. We went to the doctor's office for a blood sugar check, and her suspicion was quickly confirmed.

I grew up in a small town, so the pediatrician referred us to the endocrinologists at Riley Hospital for Children in Indianapolis. We gathered some things from home and made the two-hour drive that day. In retrospect, I am thankful this wasn't more of an urgent, emergency-level situation. I know many people have pretty traumatic diagnosis stories. But in that moment, at 12 years old, of course my mind wasn't there. My own diagnosis I was experiencing was all I knew of diabetes at that point.

My dad, my mom, and I spent the next three days learning what life would look like moving forward. It was a lot to take in. It changed our thought process on food and how we looked at exercise. We learned to count carbs and give shots. And we always carried insulin and sugar with us wherever we went from that day on.

Diabetes doesn't run in my family, and my parents didn't know of anyone who dealt with it either. I didn't have any friends with type 1. And while the doctors did an amazing job of checking in on us for the first several weeks, we were fairly isolated in this new journey.

If this is you, if you are relating personally to anything I'm saying, I just want to encourage you that you are not alone. I have been there myself, and I know it's hard. You are likely learning a ton, dealing with grief, asking loads of questions, and second guessing everything you're doing. It's all very new, and it's ok. Find your people, do your best, and give yourself grace.

More than anything, you are not alone because God is always with you—whether you experienced a diagnosis yesterday or decades ago.

Consider the story of Hagar in Genesis chapter 16. (If you've not reviewed this story in a while, it's a great read.) In short, God has promised Abram and Sarai many descendants, but that's yet to come true. So Sarai suggests her servant Hagar have a baby with Abram instead. Hagar conceives a child, Sarai starts to mistreat her, and Hagar runs away.

So there she is, pregnant and alone in the wilderness. Feeling uncertain and vulnerable, Hagar is visited by an angel of the Lord. After receiving the angel's message, she calls God "El Roi" or "the God who sees."

> She gave this name to the Lord who spoke to her: "You are the God who sees me," for she said, "I have now seen the One who sees me."
> Genesis 16:13 (NIV)

Now, I think it's important to note that God doesn't immediately fix Hagar's problem. In fact, He tells her to return to it. But He recognizes her suffering, and she knows that He sees her. And if God is with her in the wilderness, He will be with her when she returns to Sarai. She can now face her difficult situation with His presence and strength.

We can face our toughest battles and most challenging days with His presence and strength as well, knowing that God sees us too, friend. He sees everything clearly, He watches over us continually, and He is with us always. He sees us trying and He knows our hearts.

My hope and my prayer for you is this: even though there will be times of feeling totally overwhelmed with all that is diabetes, and even though you will feel frustrated with all the bobbing and lurching on these high seas, that you will personally encounter the God who sees you.

God, thank You for this reminder and perspective today. Thank You for Hagar's story and the lessons I can learn from it. In this world where things can make me feel isolated and unimportant and alone, I know You see me. Help me to remember that every day. Remind me I am made in Your image and with a purpose, and that diabetes doesn't get to define that—You do. Thank You for Your love and faithfulness. Amen.

Reading

Genesis 16, Psalm 33:18

Reflection

What does the story of Hagar show us about God? Write a short prayer on the lines provided as you remind yourself that God sees you.

_____

_____

_____

_____

_____

_____

_____

_____

thoughts + prayers

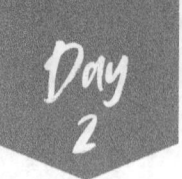

CHARTING EXPECTATIONS

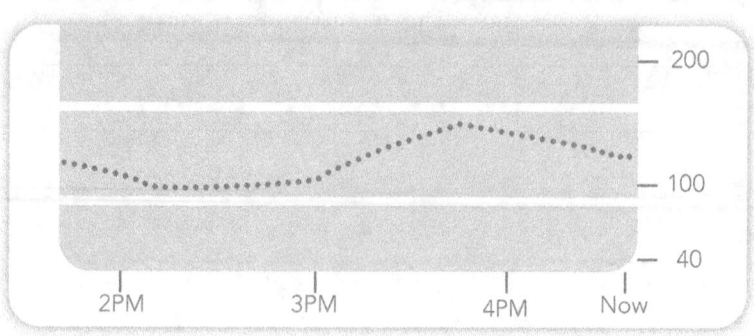

If daily life were a continuous glucose monitor (CGM) graph, this is what I expect my average day to look like. I'm a planner by default, a scheduler of all things. I can look ahead and know what we will have for dinner later in the week, when I have appointments of any kind, days our daughter has softball games, and so much more. I generally go to bed at night having a pretty sure feeling of what the next day will hold.

What's more interesting is the graph I would show you that represents my day when it's over. It would look much more like this.

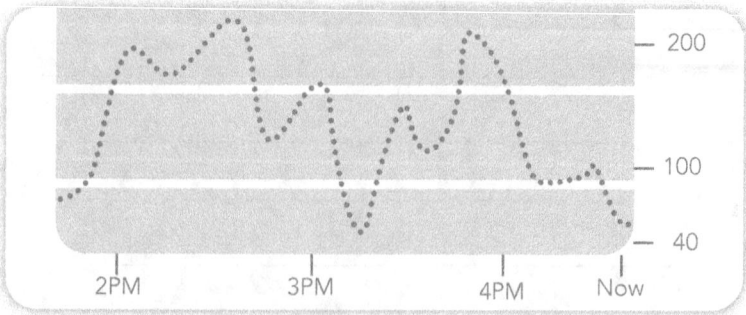

Not all that close, is it? Even though I prepare for the day, life has a way of finding its own course. An unexpected meeting is scheduled at work.

A disagreement happens with a close friend. The fridge quits working. A child gets sick. The car tire goes flat. The stuff of life can derail your day.

And of course we all deal with the diabetes stuff on top of daily life as well. You run into an issue at the pharmacy. Your blood sugar isn't cooperating and you aren't sure why. You spend what seems like hours on hold for a doctor's office or insurance representative. You experience a blood sugar low while exercising and have to stop to treat it. It's all the things.

It's the same concept in our walk with the Lord. We expect the line of what will happen in our spiritual life to be pretty straight and even. People tend to think the moment they are lifted out of the waters of baptism that the angels will sing (they do), our troubles will fade away (they don't), and life as a follower of Jesus will just be…easy (it's not).

Why do we expect that? There's nothing in the Bible that promises anything close to an easy life with no troubles. In fact, scripture tells us the opposite.

> *Consider it joy, my brothers and sisters, whenever you face trials of many kinds…*
> *James 1:2 (NIV)*

James, the brother of Jesus, tells us to find joy in our trials. Not *if* you face trials, but *when* you face trials. So if we are bound to face challenges, how do we find joy in them? His direction seems counterintuitive at first. But the answer for us is in the very next verses:

> *…because you know that the testing of your faith produces perseverance. Let perseverance finish its work so that you may be mature and complete, not lacking anything.*
> *James 1:3-4 (NIV)*

Times of trial help us grow. James is encouraging us to embrace those moments and look to God to help us grow through them.

Life doesn't always go as we plan, does it? Over time the tides can change. You can't stop the waves from coming, but you can learn to look at them through a different lens. Those waves are opportunities for you to trust and follow God, and for Him to work in your heart and mind. Remember today what Jesus told us in the gospel of John.

> In this world you will have trouble. But take heart! I have overcome the world.
> John 16:33 (NIV)

God, thank You for Your ability to see things I can't see. Thank You for the big picture of Your grand story. And thank You for using the struggles in life to shape and mold me, to bring good out of the challenge. Help me to have a big-picture perspective more often. And thank You, Jesus, that You teach me and give me this wisdom I can carry in my daily life. Thank You that You have overcome the world! Amen.

Reading

Proverbs 4:25-26, Romans 5:3-5

Reflection

What expectations do you have with diabetes? What expectations do you have of God?

How would looking at challenges through James' lens be helpful?

_____

_____

_____

_____

_____

thoughts + prayers

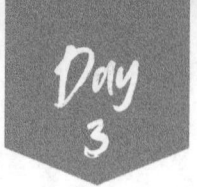

NOTHING MAKES SENSE

It had happened every week for at least a month. The hustle to get ready and out the door on Sunday morning, with two littles to check into kids church, left me low heading into worship. It was like clockwork. Around 9am my CGM was reading about 70, and I would find myself chomping on glucose gummies as everyone else was singing.

After a family joke that going to church made me low, I decided to cut back on my insulin in the morning the following week. So I ate the exact same breakfast at the exact same time (I'm nothing if not consistent), but instead of telling my pump I had eaten 46g of carbs, I entered 42g. I was thinking with that small a change I'd land around 90 or 100. Nope…204.

Of course, this made zero sense to me. But there are times literally nothing makes sense to me with this disease. I can try my best and completely win the day, and I can try my best and end up scratching my head in confusion. The uncertainty. The frustration. Sometimes nothing about diabetes seems to be logical. Even thirty years in, I still have those "I just don't get it" moments.

And all the non-food variables that affect blood sugar certainly don't help: exercise, the timing of insulin, medication interactions, changes in sleep, hormone swings, increased stress, illness, even sunburns or seasonal allergies…the list goes on.

What do you do when diabetes doesn't make sense? Do you call your doctor? Do you chat with a friend who understands? Do you just vent to anyone who will listen? Do you make adjustments in hopes of improving next time? With diabetes, every day can be a bit different. What works today may not work tomorrow or next week. (Queue the next frustration.) And we're stuck in a cycle of nothing making sense.

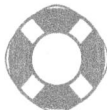

So what if we, instead of seeking answers to specific scenarios that may change over time, simply did our best with diabetes and started searching for peace in the midst of what doesn't make sense? When we face the frustrations of diabetes, our souls need the peace that surpasses all understanding (Philippians 4:7). And that peace comes only from connecting with our Heavenly Father.

Like a child wanting mommy to wrap her arms around them, like a toddler snuggling on daddy's lap, we should approach our Heavenly Father with the innocence and hope and trust of a child. His arms are ever-open wide. His lap is always available. He is our loving, comforting "Abba" Father.

> Draw near to God, and He will draw near to you.
> James 4:8 (ESV)

Lean into Him in these frustrating moments that come more often than you would like. Approach Him and He will meet you there with immeasurable peace like a river to offer every time.

Heavenly Father, I thank You today for Your peace. Your unexplainable peace in the face of what feels like chaos. And I thank You for always being available so I am able to approach You at any time. Father, there are so many days things just don't make any sense with this disease. Things happen that simply don't seem logical. At least not to me. Not in my human mind. But I know You understand everything. You see it all playing out. I ask You today to help me seek out Your lasting peace more than I search for fleeting answers. Comfort me with this peace today, God. Amen.

Reading

John 14:25-27, Romans 15:13

Reflection

What do the two passages of additional reading today tell us about the Holy Spirit and peace?

Write your thoughts or a prayer on the lines provided.

_____

_____

_____

_____

_____

_____

_____

_____

_____

_____

PEACE I LEAVE WITH YOU;
MY PEACE I GIVE TO YOU.

JOHN 14:27 (ESV)

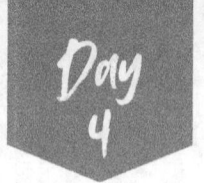

Day 4

THE WAIT

Time seems to move so slowly when we wait. We wait on little things… for our blood sugar to come up after a low, to eat when our number is too high, for prescriptions to be refilled, for CGMs to warm up. We wait on bigger things, too…for our A1c to improve, for better technology, for a different medication that works better, for an update from the doctor. And we wait for a cure.

We wait. And then we wait some more, don't we?

As a great man of faith and a man after God's own heart, King David was intimately familiar with waiting. He was only a young shepherd, the youngest of eight boys, when he was anointed to be the next king of Israel. While he waited, he became King Saul's armor bearer, conquered Goliath, and was then banished and nearly killed by Saul. He hid in the desert, lived on the run, and fought many battles. Most scholars say it was about 15 years between David being anointed and becoming king. He did his fair share of waiting.

But look what God taught him in the wait. Just read the Psalms he wrote! David is one of the most transparent and vulnerable people in the Bible about his agony in the wait, yet his heart was steadfast and set on God. He learned to trust in Him. He learned to look to Him. He learned to rely on Him. He learned to wait on Him.

> *How long, Lord? Will you forget me forever?*
> *How long will you hide your face from me?*
> *How long must I wrestle with my thoughts*
> *and day after day have sorrow in my heart?*
> *How long will my enemy triumph over me?*
> *Look on me and answer, Lord my God.*
> *Give light to my eyes, or I will sleep in death,*

> and my enemy will say, "I have overcome him,"
> and my foes will rejoice when I fall.
> But I trust in your unfailing love;
> my heart rejoices in your salvation.
> I will sing the Lord's praise,
> for he has been good to me.
> Psalm 13 (NIV)

David ended up ruling as king for 40 years, and he became known as the greatest ruler of Israel. But in his 15-year wait, God provided and protected him. God refined him through trials and missteps. And it resulted in David's amazing faith that you and I can look back on. Even today, God is reaching people through David.

Here's the key: David was anchored in God. Through it all, even with his life at risk over and over, David can still say, "for He has been good to me" (Psalm 13:6b NIV).

God is not in a hurry. He doesn't seem to mind waiting. In the quiet times when we find ourselves frustrated and waiting for answers, know that God is still at work. In these moments, our faith has the opportunity to be stretched and grown, and our relationship with God can be strengthened. So much good can come in the wait.

So what will you do while you wait? You have a choice. You can let diabetes break you down, or you can give the wait to God and allow Him to build you up. The decision is yours.

God, thank You for the example of King David, for his openness about his challenges and his continual gaze on You. Thank You for the lessons You taught Him, and for his faith that is an encouragement to me today. Help me, God, to be patient. Calm my heart as I learn more and more to trust in You. Help me to remember You are at work; help me to wait well. Help me to look forward to knowing the work You will do—the work You already have in progress. Help me to rely on You, God, as the anchor for my life. Amen.

Reading

Genesis 18:1-15 (Abraham and Sarah)
Genesis 37, 39-45 (Joseph)
John 5:1-15 (The Man at the Pool)
John 11:1-44 (Lazarus)
1 Samuel 1 (Hannah)
Luke 1:67-80 (The Long-Awaited Messiah)

Reflection

Take a moment to read another story listed above about God's people in waiting and what ultimately came of it. Then journal your thoughts about what they learned in the wait. Pray for the things God will do in you and through you in your wait.

_____
_____
_____
_____
_____
_____
_____
_____
_____

thoughts + prayers

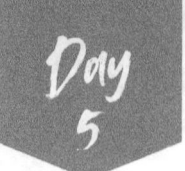

WANDERING AWAY

Have you ever just had your fill of diabetes? Have you ever wanted to throw in the towel? Have you ever thought enough is enough?

Aside from the never-ending nature of this chronic illness, all the medication and beeping and carb counting and appointments and sleep loss can sure add up to drag us down. It's no wonder people with diabetes often wander away from taking good care of themselves.

I get it. Thirty years into this relationship with diabetes now, I have definitely wanted a break (and far more than once). But here's what I know for certain: no matter how long you've faced burnout, no matter how long you've ignored your blood sugar, no matter how long it's been since you counted a single carbohydrate, it's not too late to turn around. Your health and ultimately your very life are at stake.

If you are relating to what I'm saying here, I just want to encourage you today. It's not too late to make changes. Now, you don't have to be perfect immediately. You don't have to go from zero to 100%. Burnout can make great diabetes management feel impossible. So don't focus on great. Great can be overwhelming.

Just try to do the next right thing. Focus on just that day, or even part of a day. And then do it again. Pretty soon you'll start to see a difference. And don't be down on yourself for wandering. We are prone to wander.

We are prone to wander from God as well. He knows we are. God knows His creation is pulled to drift away. This world around us closes in hard, and we walk in one direction or another away from what God would want for us. And sometimes we even intentionally wander away.

This reminds me of a parable Jesus tells in Luke chapter 15 about a boy who decided he'd be better off on his own. He took his inheritance in advance from his father, set off for another country, and ended up completely wasting it all away. Ultimately, he had no choice but to get whatever work he could, and he found himself feeding pigs. The longer he starved due to a famine in the area, the more appetizing the pig food looked to him!

Once he realized what he was doing, he decided to return home and beg for his father's forgiveness. He thought maybe, just maybe, his father would allow him to become a servant. He felt he was no longer worthy to be called his son. But as he neared his home, his father saw him from a distance. Much to the boy's surprise, his father came running toward him, threw his arms around him, and celebrated his return!

> *"For this son of mine was dead and is alive again; he was lost and is found." So they began to celebrate.*
> Luke 15:24 (NIV)

Have you ever wandered away from God like the son in this story wandered from his father? Have you ever noticed you're starting to drift? It typically happens slowly, and it takes a while to realize it most of the time. But at some point, we catch on. And when we do, it's not too late to turn around. Yes, we are prone to wander from God, but here's the good news: we can return home.

I pray that this parable is a reminder to you today that we can turn back to God if we have wandered away. I pray the incredible love and forgiveness on the part of the father in this story gives you a glimpse into the love and forgiveness of our Heavenly Father. That is the love we have available to us when we find ourselves wandering from God. He is always there with open arms to welcome a wandering soul. He will delight in celebration when His children return home.

God, I thank You for Your unending love. You love in a depth so much greater than I can understand, and I thank You for Your incredible love today. When I start to wander from You, Father, help me to realize it and return to You. Help me to know You love me all the time, and that there is nothing I can do that could separate me from Your love. Amen.

Reading

Luke 15:11-32, Romans 5:8, Romans 8:38-39, Ephesians 3:14-19

Reflection

Take some time today to read Luke 15:11-32. Consider what we can learn about God's incredible love for His children as shown through the character of the father in this parable.

thoughts + prayers

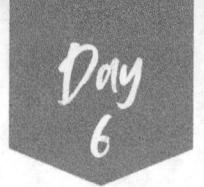

Day 6

ISOLATION

My husband and I had just walked into a restaurant for a rare mid-week date night, taking full advantage of the kids being with his parents for a couple days. As soon as we sat down, my CGM gave me a rise alert. *Doo-dle-dee-doo-dle-dee-doo!* My husband (and everyone else in the small restaurant) heard it loud and clear. He raised his eyebrows, smiled at me, and said, "It sounds like you won!"

While it may have sounded like I had just conquered the highest level in the latest video game, I wasn't exactly winning when my number was on the rise just before ordering a meal. But that's ok. I like his sense of humor and casual conversation about all the beeping I do. Everywhere I go. Regardless of who is around. So, we laughed and went on with the conversation like it was normal.

But it's not always this way. Not everyone understands. And not everyone wants to understand. It can make me feel different. Weird. Excluded. Lonely. Isolated.

People dealing with diabetes can face a host of isolating experiences. They can be judged for their choices in food, their weight, or the medical equipment visible on their bodies. They can be harassed, put down, and made fun of at work or school. It's a lot to manage, and other people notice. The beeping. The pump wearing. The insulin injecting. The finger pricking. The CGM peeking out from under the arm of a tee shirt while a little kid frowns and points and says, "What's that?!" (An innocent question, I have no doubt, but it can feel isolating.)

So how do we handle these feelings of isolation? First, we can remind ourselves we're not alone. Maybe the guy at the next table in the restaurant doesn't understand, but 10% of the world's population has been diagnosed with diabetes. That may not sound like a high

percentage, but that accounts for 537 million people in this world.* It's pretty safe to say we're not alone.

More importantly, we are not alone because God is always with us. That is a promise we can cling to. God says to His people:

> Be strong and courageous. Do not be afraid or terrified because of them, for the Lord your God goes with you; he will never leave you nor forsake you.
> Deuteronomy 31:6 (NIV)

And then God says to Joshua, Israel's new leader at the time:

> Have I not commanded you? Be strong and courageous. Do not be afraid; do not be discouraged, for the Lord your God will be with you wherever you go.
> Joshua 1:9 (NIV)

God is consistent in His message, isn't He? And He is consistently with us. We are never alone. That is a promise we can cling to, even when we feel like we are all alone out in the middle of the vast ocean and no one is with us. God is with us.

God, thank You for Your promises and Your faithfulness. Thank You that You are always with us—that nothing can separate us from Your love. Remind me of this when I feel isolated. Bring to my mind the promise that You are always with me. That You will never leave me. That You will not forsake me. Thank You, God, for Your consistent presence in my life. Amen.

*https://www.thediabetescouncil.com/how-many-people-in-the-world-have-diabetes/

Reading

Deuteronomy 31, Joshua 1, Isaiah 41:10

Reflection

Write out Romans 8:38-39 on the lines provided and pray over its comforting truths today. Return to this page when feelings of isolation start to creep in so you can be reminded you are not alone.

_____

_____

_____

_____

_____

_____

_____

_____

_____

_____

_____

_____

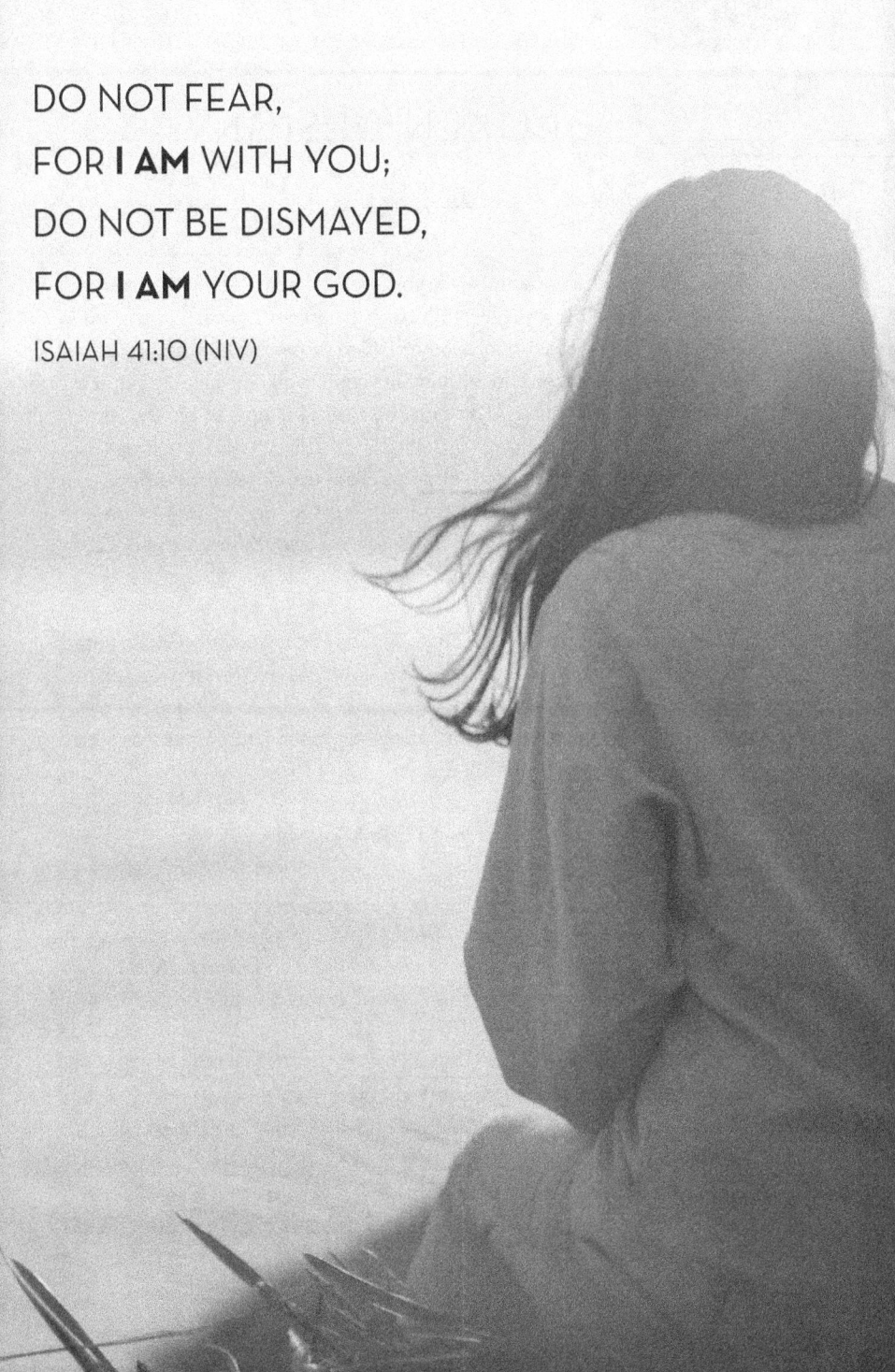

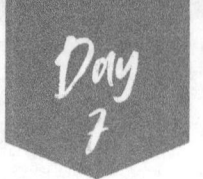

BROKEN DESIGN

Have you ever wondered why you were diagnosed with diabetes? Personally, I can't tell you why I have it. The best "guess" I have been offered is that, once upon a time, I took a medication as a kid that affected my pancreas and it ultimately quit working. Like I said, it's a guess. But we as humans like to make sense of things, so we try.

I can't tell you why someone else has diabetes either. (I sure hope you weren't expecting that.) But I can tell you this: we live in a fallen and broken world full of illness and disease. It's a tragedy, honestly, because it wasn't at all what God created.

In the very beginning of the Bible, in Genesis chapter 1, God created the heavens and the earth. He made light, sky, water, ground, plants, day and night, creatures of the water, birds of the air, animals, people… everything! It was all new and amazing—so much so that this was God's response at the end of the sixth day:

> God saw all that he had made, and it was very good.
> Genesis 1:31 (NIV)

Close your eyes and picture what Adam and Eve saw. Such a scene must have been completely and peacefully beautiful and serene. And it was, until corruption in the form of a serpent entered God's design to sink the ship.

In Genesis 3, a mere three short chapters into the beginning of the creation story, it all started to unravel. In short, the serpent showed up and started to question Eve about what God said. He convinced her to question God and eat the fruit of the only forbidden tree. Then she convinced Adam, who was there with her, to eat it too. They both sinned against God. When God confronted them about it, Eve blamed the serpent, Adam blamed Eve, and they were banished from the garden.

> So the Lord God banished him [Adam] from the Garden of Eden to work the ground from which he had been taken.
> Genesis 3:23 (NIV)

And that was it. All things hurtful, shameful, sinful, and painful entered into this world. God's precious and perfect creation was broken.

Yes, God created the universe and everything in it. But diabetes was not part of His design. There was nothing hurtful, shameful, sinful, or painful in His creation. But we now live in this fallen and broken world—and diabetes is a part of *that*.

The good news for us today is that this world won't be broken forever. God promises to restore His children to Him in a new heaven and new earth. The first part of Revelation chapter 21 tells us that God will live among us one day, that He will wipe away every tear, and that the old order of things will pass away. He will make all things new. One day it will all be perfect again. It's another beautiful picture to close our eyes and anticipate.

The other good news is that, even in this broken world, this disease doesn't define you. (We'll unpack this more on day 14, so hold onto this thought.) We can live with diabetes and still be a beautiful creation of God, fully loved by Him. God created you in His image, with a purpose and on purpose.

Let's choose to cling to what we know is true today.

Lord God, You are the creator of heaven and earth, and of each one of us. Although I live in a world filled with things You didn't intend in Your original design, I was still fearfully and wonderfully made by You. Thank You for Your design. When I start to doubt things around me and try to make sense of the things in this world, I pray You would continually point me to the truth of Your Word and Your unconditional love. Amen.

Reading

Psalm 139, Revelation 21:1-5

Reflection

Let's refresh our minds and refocus our attention by reviewing Psalm 139. Write on the lines provided what you learn from these verses about yourself and about God.

thoughts + prayers

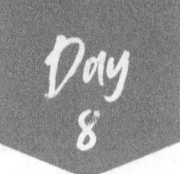

Day 8

UNANSWERED QUESTIONS

I remember it like it was yesterday. I was sitting in the bathroom, all of 12 years old, watching my mother pull insulin into the syringe. I had just been diagnosed a few weeks prior, and this was my new normal. I looked up at her through tears and asked the hard question I desperately wanted answered. Why me?

Those two simple words held so many others unspoken. What did I do to deserve an incurable disease? How could I have stopped this from happening? How would I live the rest of my days dependent on just the right amount of medication to keep me alive? What could I do to feel like my life was "normal" again? And with no one on either side of my family having type 1 diabetes, why did I suddenly have it?

It all felt so unknowable.

Mom looked back at me, shook her head, and said softly, "I don't know, sweetie. I don't know."

As I've said before, it's human nature to want answers, to search for meaning, to want to understand why. Even at age 12. But more than 30 years later, I still don't have answers to all those questions. And I bet you have some unanswered questions, too. We all do.

While you and I may not always see the answers we crave, we can still trust in the Lord. He provides for us, sustains us, and walks with us through it all. Every moment of every day. Through the known and unknown, the challenging and the simple. An often-quoted verse in Proverbs encourages us in this.

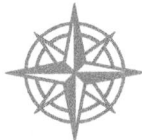

> Trust in the Lord with all your heart and lean not on your own understanding; in all your ways submit to him, and he will make your paths straight.
> Proverbs 3:5-6 (NIV)

While God may or may not reveal answers to our aching questions, this verse shows us He will guide us down the path. Sometimes we don't need answers as much as we simply need to know the next step to take. God doesn't always provide what we want, but He always provides what we need. And what we need most is Him.

God can handle your tough questions. Ask Him anything on your heart. You may not get direct or immediate answers, but you will certainly find Him there with you.

> Cast all your anxiety on him because he cares for you.
> 1 Peter 5:7 (NIV)

Lord, thank You for the promises throughout Scripture that You are my provider and sustainer, and that You are with me always. Thank You for the invitation to turn to You any time I feel unsure and uncertain. If I'm fully honest, there are times I struggle to trust in You, especially when I don't understand something. Please help me want You more than I want answers. Please remind me that You are enough, and I don't always need solutions as much as I simply need You. Amen.

Reading

Psalm 13

Reflection

What burning questions do you have? What has plagued your mind, coming up time and again with no resolution? Write it down on the lines provided. Speak it aloud. Lay those mysteries at the feet of Jesus. They aren't mysteries to Him.

_____

_____

_____

_____

_____

_____

_____

_____

_____

_____

_____

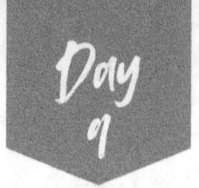

Day 7

A THANKFUL HEART

"What are the three inventions that have impacted your life the most?" That was the question from our dinnertime conversation starters. Our nine-year-old daughter immediately offered up, "the bicycle!" Of course. It was top of mind, as she had just come in from riding it to eat dinner.

Our four-year-old son continued to be lost in his macaroni and cheese, so my husband (the realist) said, "If we were all to be honest, we would say things like electricity, indoor plumbing, and running water."

I mean, he wasn't wrong. And while I don't like to imagine my life without those things, I had something else in mind. "I would say insulin, my pump, and my CGM," I said. "They all work together to basically keep me alive."

Like electricity, indoor plumbing, and running water, there was a time (not all that long ago) when people lived without many technological advances in the world of diabetes. Insulin wasn't discovered until 1921. Blood sugar meters weren't around until the 1970s, and even then they were only in doctors' offices and hospitals. The first insulin pump came into existence in the 1970s as well, but it was more like carrying a toaster oven strapped over your entire back. It was so huge it was never put on the market because it was completely impractical.

Today we have monitors the size of a quarter that measure blood sugar levels every five minutes. We have pumps smaller than your hand that just clip on wherever you put them. We have smart-dosing insulin pens. Our devices can "talk" to each other and work together for us. And much more. I think it's safe to say we have come a long way!

We have so much to be thankful for, friend. And we have so many people behind the scenes to be thankful for as well. They are paving the way

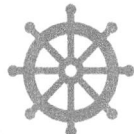

for us and for future generations. We can be thankful to God for them. Every step of progress made toward a healthier life is a gift from God. He works through those in the medical community as they come together to provide better treatment options and better quality of life for those dealing with diabetes.

Consider these words of the Psalmist:

> Shout for joy to the Lord, all the earth.
> Worship the Lord with gladness;
> come before him with joyful songs.
> Know that the Lord is God.
> It is he who made us, and we are his;
> we are his people, the sheep of his pasture.
> Enter his gates with thanksgiving
> and his courts with praise;
> give thanks to him and praise his name.
> For the Lord is good and his love endures forever;
> his faithfulness continues through all generations.
> Psalm 100 (NIV)

God, thank You for giving us life. I thank You today for the many men and women who have progressed the care of those with diabetes. And I pray today for those who will follow in their footsteps. May they seek You in all they do. May those You created and sustain who live with diabetes experience a healthier life because of Your work through the medical community. Through all the hardships and challenges those dealing with diabetes face, help us all to live with a grateful and thankful heart. Amen.

Reading

Psalm 136:1, James 1:17, 1 Thessalonians 5:16-18

Reflection

Choose one of the three additional readings above to write on the lines provided. Read over it multiple times and allow your heart to anchor in truth and gratitude.

thoughts + prayers

Day 10

PERMISSION TO MOURN

I set out on a morning walk, my CGM on my arm, phone in my pocket, and a juice box in my hand. (If I needed to treat a low, I'd temporarily look like a four-year-old child. But at least it's easy to carry, so that's what I do.) As I started out, I allowed my mind to drift back to a conversation I had with my father.

Shortly after the 30-year anniversary of my diabetes diagnosis, I asked my dad if he remembered anything about that day. He closed his eyes and nodded his head. "I sure do," he said. "That was the day I lost my little girl."

He went on to talk about how I, being twelve years old at the time, grew up very quickly after being diagnosed with type 1. He remembers me checking my own blood sugar, taking insulin by myself, and letting him know if I needed some juice. He wasn't given a warning or any prior notice, but he watched his daughter's childhood get cut short. He felt it slip away quickly, and he mourned the loss.

As people with diabetes, or as close friends and family members of someone with diabetes, we experience a unique sense of loss with this life-long illness. We suffer the loss of health, of course, but also a loss of innocence when a child is diagnosed. The loss of the easiness of life as we knew it. The loss of certain freedoms. The loss of spontaneity and flexibility, to an extent. The loss of predictability and feelings of certainty and stability. The loss of control we once thought we had.

We experience very real losses with diabetes, and it's ok to mourn these things. It's ok to grieve.

Grief flooded the scene in John chapter 11 when word came to Jesus that His close friend Lazarus was ill and dying. Mary and Martha, sisters of

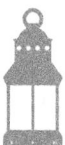

Lazarus, were also close to Jesus. And when they ultimately brought Him to the tomb where Lazarus lay, Jesus was moved to tears. He wept not only because Lazarus had died, although He knew he would rise again, but also because He was sad for His close friends and the people in the crowd who were mourning. He was sympathetic and compassionate toward them, being emotionally present. He saw their grief and met them right where they were. Right in the middle of their heartbreak and loss.

He went on to perform one of the most outrageous and amazing miracles of all—raising a man who had been dead for four days. But before doing so, Jesus Himself grieved. And we can grieve over our losses as well. We cannot possibly go wrong when we follow the example of Jesus.

> *Rejoice with those who rejoice; mourn with those who mourn.*
> *Romans 12:15 (NIV)*

God, thank You for the humanity of Jesus—that although He was fully God, He was fully human, and He experienced a full range of emotions including mourning and grief. Thank You that I have a Savior who understands the experiences I face. And thank You, God, for the comfort and sympathy You provide in these times. Thank You for Your Word that encourages me and reminds me of Your goodness and nearness. I pray You would comfort me in the losses I experience. Help me to feel Your presence. Amen.

Reading

John 11:1-44, 2 Corinthians 4:8-10, Psalm 46:1

Reflection

There are several instances in this story that show us the character of Jesus. Read through the full story of Jesus raising Lazarus (John 11:1-44) and write your thoughts or a prayer about what this story reveals to you about Jesus.

_____

_____

_____

_____

_____

_____

_____

_____

_____

_____

_____

_____

_____

thoughts + prayers

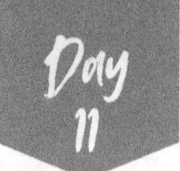

Day 11

THE BEST MEDICINE

Before 1921, a diabetes diagnosis was a death sentence. Then a surgeon and his assistant learned how to extract insulin from the pancreas of a dog. And they kept a different dog with diabetes alive with that extraction. *(Side note: This is yet another reason I think dogs are "man's best friend.")*

That same year, insulin was developed from the pancreas of cattle. And the year following that, a 14-year-old boy received the first ever human injection of insulin that ultimately dropped his severely hyperglycemic blood sugar down into normal range.

Word spread around the world quickly. There was a Nobel Prize awarded, large scale insulin manufacturers started production, the first synthetic insulin was produced, and the rest is history.*

For those with diabetes, this changed the entire trajectory of life's course. It was literally saving lives. It was the best medicine ever.

Those of us with diabetes need medication to survive, yes. But God provides the medicine we need for our souls—an everlasting cure that will carry us into eternity.

Long, long ago, God, in all His infinite knowledge and wisdom, already had a plan. A plan of redemption for all of God's people. He knew that not one of us was or would be without sin, and that meant we would all ultimately die and be separated from Him for all of eternity. He just couldn't let that happen to His own creation that He loves so dearly.

So one day, more than 2,000 years ago, He put His plan into action. God sent Jesus, while we still actively lived in sin, to take our place and pay

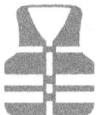

for our sin. To die on our behalf. To cover us so we could be with God in eternity together. It's a gift of life. Eternal life.

Now, we each have the opportunity to call on the name of the Lord and be saved. We can confess Jesus as our Savior and ask Him to lead our lives. Then, having been justified through faith, we have peace with God through our Lord Jesus Christ. And we can know with certainty what the Apostle Paul tells us in Romans.

> For I am convinced that neither death nor life, neither angels nor demons, neither the present nor the future, nor any powers, neither height nor depth, nor anything else in all creation, will be able to separate us from the love of God that is in Christ Jesus our Lord.
> Romans 8:38-39 (NIV)

Do you know Jesus? The gift of God is eternal life through Him. Friend, Jesus changes the entire course of life as we know it. Not only is He literally saving lives—He is saving souls! And if you don't yet know Him, He's waiting for you. He is the best medicine ever.

Lord God, thank You for the amazing discovery of insulin that helps keep me alive today to carry out Your will here on earth. And thank You for all the technologies that have come along since then. But most of all, Lord, thank You for carrying out such a selfless rescue mission to save me and offer me eternal life with You. What an incredible gift! One I never earned, don't deserve, and couldn't repay. But You love with a depth I will likely never understand. And so, I simply and humbly thank You. Amen.

*More details at: https://diabetes.org/blog/history-wonderful-thing-we-call-insulin

Reading

John 3:16-21, and several verses paraphrased in paragraphs 6-8: Romans 8:23, 6:23, 5:8, 10:9, 5:1, 8:1, and 8:38-39

Reflection

The verses in John 3:16-21 contain some of the most often quoted verses in the Bible. But I pray today you read it with fresh eyes. As you do, consider your walk with the Lord. Is it just beginning? Write a prayer for God to guide you on this new journey with Him. Is it familiar for you to walk with God? Write a prayer for Him to give you fresh eyes and to renew your mind as you continue on with Him. Above all, give Him thanks for Jesus and His love today.

_____

_____

_____

_____

_____

_____

_____

_____

_____

_____

_____

LIGHT HAS COME
INTO THE WORLD.

JOHN 3:19 (NIV)

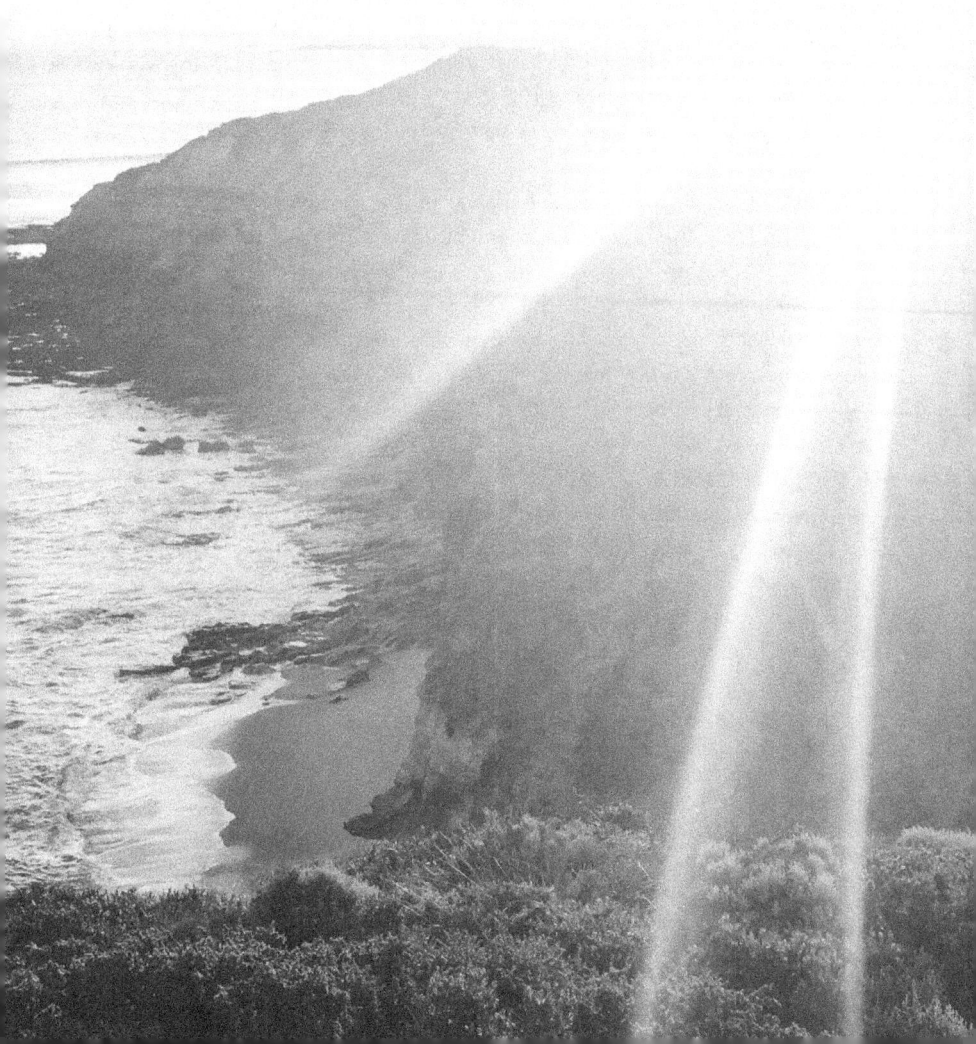

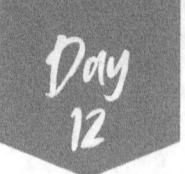

THE CARBS IN HUMBLE PIE

I woke that morning to a 100 mg/dL reading on my CGM. Perfect! My breakfast didn't cause a spike in my numbers. My afternoon walk was a piece of cake. No pun intended. And the pizza I ate for dinner? Zero highs and zero lows. I went to bed with a reading of 130. What a day!

Ok. Not all these things happened in one *actual* day that I can remember. But when these kinds of things do happen, I'm on top of the world! I feel better physically and I tend to feel super proud. I've conquered managing diabetes and I'm all puffed up with pride.

But the next day, I'll wake to a high alarm because of a pump site failure. I'll get a call that there's an insurance issue with a medication refill. My go-to meal that never spikes my numbers will send me into the 200s. Then, when I don't know the carb count for a meal out, I'll dose too much, and my sugars will plummet. I dare not even exercise! My head will hurt and I'm going to feel super tired. It's like living in the eye of the storm, and you don't know what will hurl toward you next—or when. Do you have those days too?

Honestly, do you know what I think my biggest overall issue is between these two types of days? My perspective. On good days, I typically want to take all the credit for all the good things that happened. While there isn't anything wrong with being thankful and happy with the day, if I'm not careful it can make me feel self-righteous and prideful over time. As if other people who don't have these days must not be trying because just look what I have accomplished with this major victory all on my own. (Ugh...how it hurts my heart to admit that!)

And on the hard day, I want to blame everyone and everything else. But the hard day is going to come, isn't it? And it will yank the rug right out from underneath me, as sure as the world. I'll soon be eating a big ol' heaping helping of humble pie.

So how can I avoid this?

I must become and stay humble. I'm not to take full credit for something, even if I did have a hand in it. I'm not to brag about my accomplishments. And I'm not to feel boastful about my successes or look down on others who don't share the same experience. I'm to do nothing out of selfishness, but consider others instead. The Apostle Paul reminds me of this.

> *Do nothing out of selfish ambition or vain conceit. Rather, in humility value others above yourselves, not looking to your own interests but each of you to the interests of the others.*
> *Philippians 2:3-4 (NIV)*

James, the brother of Jesus, also gives us hope when we are humble. He said:

> *Humble yourselves before the Lord and He will lift you up.*
> *James 4:10 (NIV)*

The process of being humbled feels a little like skidding down sandpaper. I just don't like it. It means I was wrong. *(Ouch!)* But that's just my flesh reacting in full to its own discomfort. It's no fun.

But when we endure, God raises us up. When we humble ourselves, we are in a position to become more and more like Jesus. We can link arms with our Heavenly Father and allow Him to transform us step by step into the likeness of His Son. And isn't that what it's all about? In the beautiful words of John the Baptist, "He must become greater; I must become less" (John 3:30 NIV).

God, thank You for Your Word and for Your guidance. Thank You for loving and caring for me so much that You provided instruction for my life through Your Word. I pray You would teach me to humble myself. Remind me not to take credit and feel prideful, but to count on You every day for Your help managing my diabetes. Remind me to thank You on the good days and pray for Your endurance and wisdom on the hard days. Thank You for the humility of Jesus as my example. Amen.

Reading

Proverbs 16:18, John 3:22-36, James 4:6-10 & 13-17

Reflection

Diabetes has a way of humbling us all from time to time. What benefits are there from being humble? How can humility help you remain anchored in God? Read the additional verses suggested above and write down your thoughts or a prayer about humility.

_____

_____

_____

_____

_____

_____

_____

_____

_____

_____

_____

thoughts + prayers

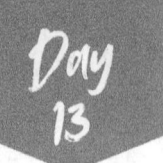

Day 13

A CALL TO PRAYER

When I saw my friend's name on my phone as it rang, I immediately knew what the call was about. She had shared with me a few days prior that she thought her daughter may have type 1. She had been working with doctors to be sure. When she called that day, she had just learned that the labs were in, and her daughter needed to be taken to the hospital.

It immediately took me back to my own diagnosis. I remember my drive to the hospital. I remember my mom telling me everything would be ok. I even remember the outfit I wore. It's etched in my memory. And with this phone call, I knew she and her daughter were about to have a very similar car ride.

Her daughter is on a sports team with mine. They were the first two people we met at my daughter's first practice. I remember the two girls buddying up to play catch, and the mom chatting with me like we were old friends. It filled my heart. Fast forward almost a year later, and my heart was aching for what they were going through.

I listened as she talked through her shock as she drove home from work to prepare for the hospital stay. It was like she was in a fog. She said it didn't even feel real. I told her I would check in with her, and I assured her I would be praying for her and for her daughter.

I felt like it was all I could do, although what I really wanted to do was to fix it for them. I wanted to take it away. I was heartbroken to know that an innocent child was sick with a chronic illness, and I felt helpless in the situation. Prayer was the best thing I could think of. So that's what I did.

As Christians, diabetes or not, we should always pray. That should be our first help, not our last resort. James reminds us of this.

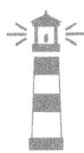

> *Is anyone among you suffering? Let him pray. Is anyone cheerful? Let him sing praise. Is anyone among you sick? Let him call for the elders of the church, and let them pray over him, anointing him with oil in the name of the Lord.*
> James 5:13-14 (ESV)

James points us to prayer whether we are struggling, happy, or ill. In other words, whatever the circumstance, we are to pray. He goes on to say in verse 16 that, "The prayer of a righteous person has great power as it is working."

Prayer literally was the best thing I could do for my friend as she entered this storm of life. Prayer is how we provide ultimate care for those we know and love, by lifting them up to the ultimate Healer of our minds, bodies, and souls.

Although prayer doesn't guarantee a solution, particularly the solution we may want at the time, it does invite God to walk with us. And there is a unique kind of healing that happens simply in sensing God's presence.

Father, thank You for the power of prayer. Thank You that You want and desire communication and relationship with me. Today I pray You would help me to make prayer my first help and not my last resort. Help me to replace worry and anxiety with prayer to You, the ultimate Healer. Amen.

Reading

Psalm 34:15, Philippians 4:6, 1 Thessalonians 5:17

Reflection

Who in your life needs prayer today? They may or may not be facing a medical diagnosis, but a hardship or challenge of some kind. How can you lift them up to the ultimate Healer? Write your prayer on the lines provided.

_____

_____

_____

_____

_____

_____

_____

_____

_____

_____

_____

thoughts + prayers

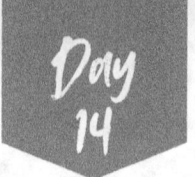

IDENTITY

———————

Am I feeling nervous or is my blood sugar low?
How many carbs are in this salad? sandwich? cookie?
Did I give myself insulin for lunch today?
Is my CGM reading accurately?
When is my next doctor appointment again?
Should I exercise now or this afternoon?
Is this headache a sign that my blood sugar is high?
Will my prescription be ready in time?
How will I pay for my medical supplies?
What does my meter say?
What does my pump say?
What will my friend say?

Diabetes can sure feel consuming. Constant questions and day-to-day thoughts can ping pong through our heads, hijacking our day and keeping us from focusing fully on other parts of our lives. It can completely take over if we let it. It can feel like it's the biggest part of our lives because it affects so many areas of our lives. Almost like it's our identity. But it isn't.

Your diagnosis is not your identity. Read that again. And you are not a diabetic. You are a child of God who is living with diabetes. Do you see the difference? It's subtle, but it's an important distinction.

So what is your identity? God created it when He created you, before you were ever born. He designed you on purpose and for a purpose, in His image, and dearly loved. Not one shred of God's design or love for you changed when you received your diagnosis. Not one. He made you, and you are His. Your identity remains the same, diabetes or not, as a precious and treasured child of God.

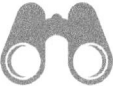

> Before I formed you in the womb I knew you, before you were born I set you apart.
> Jeremiah 1:5 (NIV)

This Word of God came to Jeremiah, a prophet of the Old Testament. What a beautiful picture of God's intentionality and love and purpose. We are merely five verses into the book of Jeremiah when we read these life-giving words. God encouraged Jeremiah early on in his ministry. He knew Jeremiah would endure challenge, conflict, and great hardship during his forty years as a prophet. Jeremiah needed to be reminded up front that he was created with a purpose and identity. And God provided just what he needed.

Like Jeremiah, you also bear a unique purpose and identity. Part of that includes your diagnosis. God knew you would have this illness. Why? That's something only He can reveal to you in His time.

Until then, allow these reassuring words of Scripture to wash over you today. Reframe your thoughts and renew your mind in this truth. Take time for prayer that God would offer you reassurance in your true identity in Him.

Heavenly Father, You are my creator and sustainer, and You sustain me with such love and intentionality. Thank You for giving me my identity in You. This chronic illness can drag me down and beat me up, and it can become easy to believe the lie that my identity is found in this never-ending disease. I need renewing, Lord. Help me with my perspective, renew my mind, and reframe my thoughts to fully grasp my true identity as Your dearly loved child. Amen.

Reading

The creation story in Genesis 1, Psalm 139:13-16, Galatians 3:23-29

Reflection

What does it mean to you to be a child of God? How can the encouraging reminder of Jeremiah 1:5 help you focus your thoughts today? Write a prayer of gratitude for your true identity.

YOUR WORKS ARE **WONDERFUL**,
I KNOW THAT FULL WELL.

PSALM 139:14 (NIV)

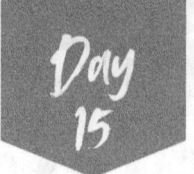

EMBRACE THE MYSTERY

As I write this devotion, my blood sugar is hovering just over 200. This isn't typical for me after a dinner that I've eaten probably twenty times before. I've already corrected with insulin, and I'm now playing the waiting game for my number to come back down into range.

Blood sugars can react differently because of so many things. It can be hard to pin down exactly what caused the deviation. Was it a lack of activity? Was it hormonal? Was it my stress level? Was there an air bubble in the tubing of my pump? It could be any one of an enormous list of things, and I may honestly never know which one.

Sometimes in life we don't understand why, and sometimes that's hard for me. I tend to be a logical person. I believe in cause and effect. But tonight, I will just deal with it the best I can and get through it here shortly. Tonight, I will embrace the mystery.

People in Bible times had to embrace the mystery, too—often in much bigger ways. And sometimes they didn't understand why either. Take the story of Joshua leading the Israelites to capture Jericho, for example. God tells Joshua to have the Israelites march around the city in silence one time each day for six days and then, on the seventh day, they are to march around it seven times and shout. Then the walls will fall and the city will be theirs.

Now, I don't know much about the inner workings of battles fought and won in Old Testament days, but I do know one thing: this was not a common battle plan. Do you think the people marching around the city day after day had a clear picture of why they were doing what they were doing? Although God told Joshua the plan ahead of time, there's nothing in the text that shows Joshua relaying the full plan to the Israelites up front. They had to go with it, trust Joshua (whom they knew was talking to God), and see it through. It took faith.

And so, the faithful people marched quietly. They saw the strong walls all around the city as they walked along day after day. What do you suppose they were thinking? Whatever it was, they obviously had enough faith in Joshua and God to carry out a plan that made very little sense.

And on the seventh day, when they had marched around the city a seventh time, Joshua gave the order to shout. The priests blew their trumpets, the people's voices rang out, and the walls of Jericho crumbled right before their eyes.

I like to imagine in that moment that Joshua remembered the first thing God said to him when He initially gave this order:

> *See, I have delivered Jericho into your hands…*
> Joshua 6:2 (NIV)

I point out this verse because God spoke that to Joshua in the past tense before Israel marched around the city even once. He knew how it would end before it began. Nothing is a mystery to our all-seeing, all-knowing, all-powerful God. He sees things with a greater perspective than we can.

God doesn't usually explain Himself ahead of time (or ever). The gospel itself is a mystery, according to Paul in Ephesians chapter 6. But Paul obviously embraced the mysteries woven through the gospel, as he continued to preach and reach people with the news of Christ.

Also, the Old Testament prophets would never have guessed that the fulfillment of the prophecies they were given would come by God Himself entering this world as an infant.

Sometimes it isn't about figuring it out, but letting go and choosing to trust. Even when you can't yet see the full picture, God can work through you to accomplish great things. Humbly submit to His will, walk in faith, and embrace the mystery.

God, I love Bible stories of faith. And these people had some incredible faith that You did incredible things with. I admit, sometimes when I can't see the full picture or understand the reason behind something, I don't want to do it. When things don't make sense, I tend to shy away. God, I pray that You would keep me from drifting away from You when I don't understand. Help me to have faith in You and Your plan regardless of what I can see in the moment. Amen.

Reading

Joshua 6, Ephesians 6:18-20

Reflection

Is there something that is a mystery to you? What can you not quite figure out? Write a prayer today that God would walk with you through the mystery, and that you would remain anchored in Him even in the unknown.

_____

_____

_____

_____

_____

_____

_____

thoughts + prayers

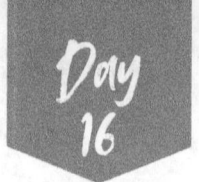

Day 16

VACATION DAYDREAMS

I pulled up in my friend's driveway on a beautiful, sunny fall morning. We loaded her family's bags into the back of my van, and I asked, "Do you have your tickets? Do you have your IDs? And do you have all the diabetes supplies for your son in a carry-on bag?" She answered yes to all of the above, and we drove off en route to the airport.

They were headed to a beach to visit some family for a week of down time, relaxation, walking along the shoreline, and all the wonderful things a vacation has to offer. I couldn't help but think, as I drove back home after wishing them well, that I would dearly love to pack up my diabetes in a suitcase and send it off for a week's vacation. I would gladly pay for the ticket! It's been 30 years now, diabetes and me, and it has never taken a week off. Not a single day. Not a single hour.

How can we, those of us who deal with diabetes day in and day out, keep our heads about ourselves when there is never a slowdown, let alone a break? Diabetes doesn't go on vacation. It literally never stops—even when we sleep. How can we keep perspective in the face of something that needs constant attention and never goes away?

I'm preaching to myself just as much as anyone else as I continue, but let's look at the example of the Apostle Paul. Now, I will admit this up front: any time I consider my life in light of his example, I can't even explain how short I measure up. But let's look into this anyway because he can teach us so much.

Paul is a guy who faced some ongoing hardship for sure. You may recall he was beaten multiple times, stoned and left for dead, thrown in jail, shipwrecked, placed under house arrest, and faced multiple assassination plots. (Ok...my non-vacationing diabetes pales in comparison already. Yours too?) Then, just a couple years before he died, Paul found himself in a prison in Rome where he penned the book of Philippians. Before closing his writing of this heartfelt letter, Paul says:

> I have learned to be content whatever the circumstances. I know what it is to be in need, and I know what it is to have plenty. I have learned the secret of being content in any and every situation, whether well fed or hungry, whether living in plenty or in want. I can do all this through him who gives me strength. Philippians 4:11-13 (NIV)

Read that last sentence again. Christ is the key. Paul says his contentment, regardless of circumstance, is due to the strength provided to him by Jesus. He has certainly experienced a full range of circumstances in his life, and he is simply sold out to Christ. No matter what it means for him. No matter what.

Are you so sold out for Christ that all else pales in comparison? Are you so on mission with Jesus that the things of life don't challenge your contentment? Are you so anchored in Christ that no wave can cast you adrift? Is Jesus your source of strength?

This is a tall, tall order, friend. And, like I said earlier, I'm preaching to myself here. Full transparency: this isn't something I do well. If you've got contentment down, let me know your secret. But for now, the rest of us, myself included, can humbly pray our way through it.

God, thank You for the example of Paul. For his transformation, for his contentment, and for his wisdom shared in the book of Philippians that we get to read even today. This chronic illness is a nagging condition that needs my constant attention. But today, Lord, I pray You will provide me an eternal perspective. I pray You will provide me strength to persevere, as You did for Paul. I pray I will become more and more sold out for You so that all else pales in comparison. Amen.

Reading

1 Timothy 6:6-7, 2 Corinthians 4:16-18, 12:9-10

Reflection

Take a look at the verses above from 1 Timothy and 2 Corinthians, two other books of the Bible penned by Paul. What consistencies do you see between those verses and the ones we studied from Philippians today? Write your thoughts and a prayer for contentment on the lines provided.

thoughts + prayers

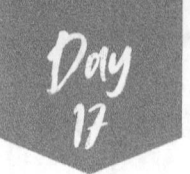

BATTLE WEARY

Diabetes has a way of exhausting people. The constant ups and downs, the additional health-related decisions, and the toll it takes on our bodies make it such a challenge. We become weary from the battle. And it's not just you and me...studies around the world have documented it.

According to the CDC, "If you get less than seven hours of sleep per night regularly, diabetes will be harder to manage."* They go on to list seven specific heightened health risk factors for those with diabetes, all connected to lack of sleep. Anyone out there struggle to get solid sleep regularly? Does it sometimes feel like diabetes makes it harder to get uninterrupted sleep? Me too.

After a 2011 UK study, the lead author said, "People who have a hard time controlling their blood glucose levels have a greater risk of complications. They have a reduced quality of life. And they have a reduced life expectancy."** Well, that's certainly heavy enough to weigh on us all. *(Ok. I think I'm done reading online articles for now.)*

The fact is the struggle is real. We will feel fatigue and burnout from trying to manage this disease well. We battle diabetes every hour of every day. It's like a storm that never stops. But even though it's hard, it's a battle worth fighting—it's a fight for life itself.

At the same time, we are also fighting a spiritual battle every day. We have a very real enemy who loves to lie to us. He delights in our frustration and fatigue over this disease. He thrives on our discouragement and depression when we are just plain worn out with it. His ultimate goal is that we slip and fall hard.

But he is stopped in his tracks when we connect with our Almighty God. He trembles at the thought of someone with even the weakest of faith

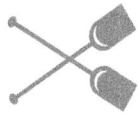

on his knees in prayer. This battle—the battle for our health and our lives—ultimately belongs to the Lord. Take it to Him in prayer.

And when we are just so exhausted with it all that we don't even know what to pray, the Spirit intercedes. The book of Romans explains.

> *In the same way, the Spirit helps us in our weakness. We do not know what we ought to pray for, but the Spirit himself intercedes for us through wordless groans.*
> Romans 8:26 (NIV)

God provides so well for us that He provides the Spirit to pray for us when we can't pray for ourselves. What a good, good, loving, caring Heavenly Father.

God, thank You for Your Spirit. Thank You for knowing what I need even before I need it. Thank You for providing so incredibly well. Father, today I pray that in moments of fatigue and frustration and burnout that You would pull me in close. Hold me tight. Keep me from the evil one. Hear my prayer today, God. You know me, You know my needs, and You see me. I pray today that You provide in ways only You can. Amen.

---

*https://www.cdc.gov/diabetes/library/features/diabetes-sleep.html
**https://www.diabetes.co.uk/news/2011/May/poor-sleep-raises-diabetic-insulin-levels,-according-to-study-99880077.html

Reading

Ephesians 6:10-20, Matthew 11:28, James 4:7

Reflection

What is your prayer today? What is the hardest part of this battle for you? Where do you need God to step in? Take it all to Him. Every bit of it. And if you don't know the first thing to pray, that's ok too. Simply sit in silence and cry out to our loving Father God for His Spirit to intercede.

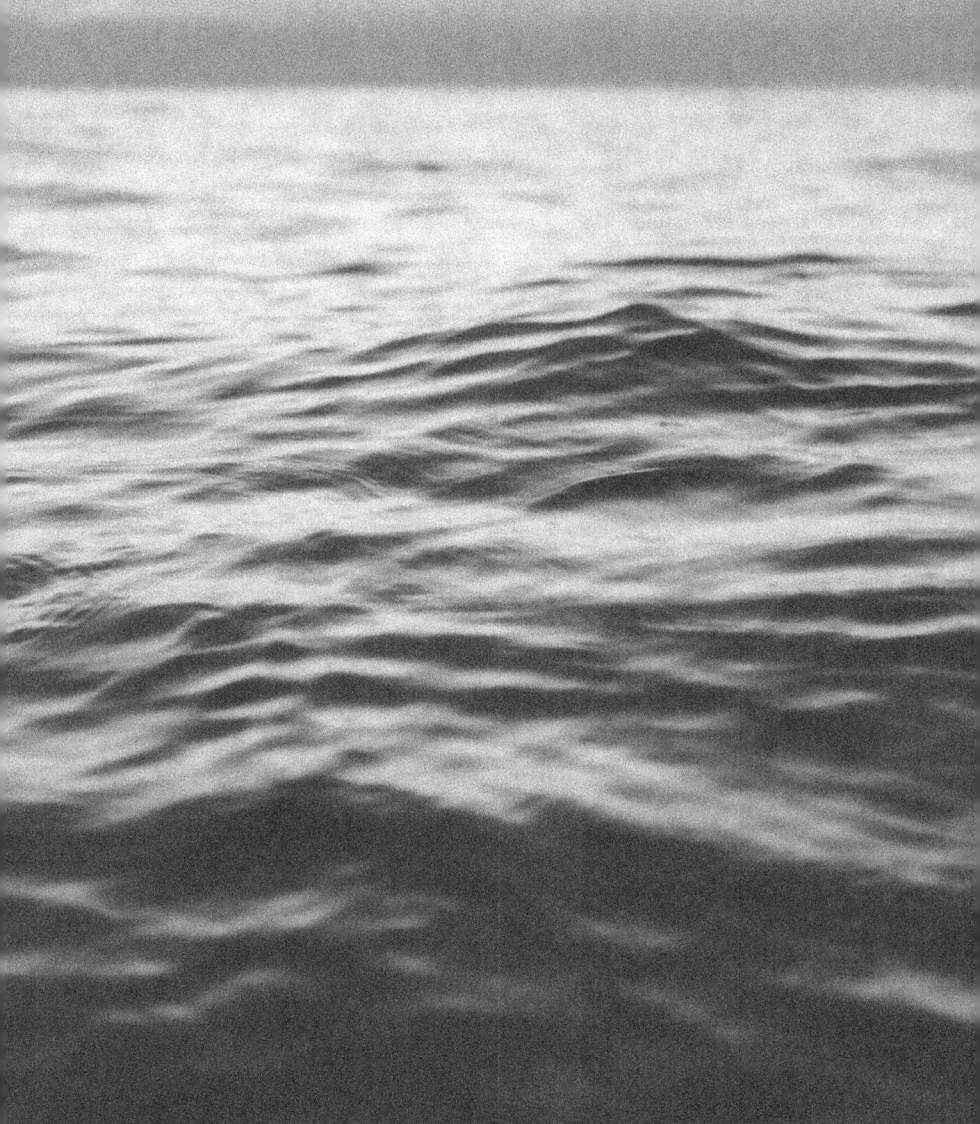

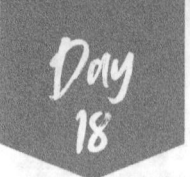

SHEER MAGNITUDE

Changing my continuous glucose monitor every ten days means I go through 36 sensors a year.

Switching out my pump supplies every three days, I go through 121 changes a year.

If I were using a meter to test my blood sugar, say, four times a day, that adds up to 1,460 test strips a year. Over 30 years, as long as I've had diabetes now, that's 43,800 test strips. If you lined them all up end to end, they would span from Sacramento to New York! Ok, they wouldn't actually reach that far (those things are tiny), but at the very least they would make an enormous pile on the floor.

The sheer magnitude of things people with diabetes need is astounding, and we've yet to touch on insulin, needles, adhesive, alcohol prep wipes, some form of fast acting sugar to correct lows…the list goes on and on. I'm sure this isn't news to you.

But no matter how overwhelming diabetes may seem, God's magnitude is greater. He shows us that nothing is too big for Him.

Think for a moment of the true magnitude of God. We don't have to look far to find evidence of it. We can see the magnitude of God in His creation. In its size and beauty. In the order of His world. In His immense creativity. In His great attention to the smallest of details and the inner workings of all He created in this incredible system of life that He spoke into existence.

> The earth is the Lord's, and everything in it,
> the world, and all who live in it;
> Psalm 24:1 (NIV)

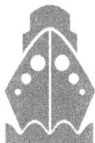

And not only did He create it, but He also sustains it. He holds everything together. That song all the cool kids have been singing for years is true: He really does hold the whole world in His hands. That's present tense on purpose. He continuously holds us.

I encourage you today to take a walk, find a park, go on a hike, sit on a bench, or rest on the porch. Take in the *magnitude* of God. See the calm water of a lake, feel a gentle breeze, and hear the sound of nature. Forget everything else, even for just a few moments, and simply dwell on the visible evidence of God all around you.

Remember as you wander and wonder, this same God dwells within us as believers in Christ when He gifts us the Holy Spirit. I'm not convinced I will ever fully understand that, but it reminds me of the vast nature of God nonetheless. And with that, I can simply be in awe.

> *For in him all things were created: things in heaven and on earth, visible and invisible, whether thrones or powers or rulers or authorities; all things have been created through him and for him. He is before all things, and in him all things hold together. Colossians 1:16-17 (NIV)*

God, You are our creator God who made the world from nothing. Thank You for Your design, for Your creativity, for Your order, and for Your intention. And You constantly sustain it all. Help me today, God, to simply sit in awe of You. Help me to enjoy Your creation and the wonder of Your magnitude. Thank You for the opportunity today to simply worship You in this way. Amen.

Reading

Psalm 19, Hebrews 1:1-4

Reflection

Use the lines provided today to capture your thoughts as you experience God's creation in nature. Write a prayer giving thanks to Him for it all.

_____

_____

_____

_____

_____

_____

_____

_____

_____

_____

_____

_____

thoughts + prayers

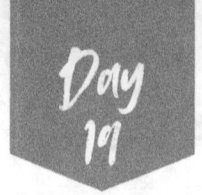

Day 19

BECOMING INTERRUPTIBLE

I glanced quickly at the clock. "Ok, kids—time to go! Let's all use the bathroom and get our shoes on," I instructed. We had fifteen minutes to get to the last day of summer camp. Driving would take ten of those minutes, and, if I'm being honest, getting the kids into the van would probably take the other five.

As I hurriedly followed my own instructions, I promptly snagged the tube to my insulin pump and pulled it straight out of my body. I was instantly annoyed. I stood there in the bathroom with my eyes closed and lips pursed, holding the dislodged tubing in my fist. I took a slow, deep breath.

Now we will be late for sure. The kids aren't listening and getting ready as I asked anyway—they're fighting about their shoes for some reason. And I now have a ten-minute job ahead of me to change everything out for my pump to work again. Of course. Why do things like this happen when I need to be somewhere? Interruptions only seem to pop up when I'm busy.

Have you been there, too? Something like this happens in a split second, and negativity floods my thoughts. Interruptions are like my kryptonite.

Interruptions happened to Jesus, too. Being the Son of God, He was certainly in high demand. And to complete His incredible mission in only three short years of ministry, He was undoubtedly busy. Yet, He was remarkably interruptible.

There was even a time when Jesus was interrupted—while He was already dealing with an interruption! Jesus was teaching to a large crowd when Jairus, a local leader in the synagogue, approached Him and begged Jesus to raise his daughter back to life. Jesus agreed, and He and His disciples left on their way to his house to heal her. On their way, a woman in the crowd who was desperate for healing reached out to touch Jesus' garments to be healed.

What I find interesting about this story is, not only that Jesus dealt with interruption on top of interruption, but also that he chose to take the time. In Mark's account of the woman in need of healing, he says:

> *Then the woman, knowing what had happened to her, came and fell at his feet and, trembling with fear, told him the whole truth.*
> Mark 5:33 (NIV)

Just how long do you imagine telling "the whole truth" might take? And what was Jairus doing while all this was going on, outside of longing for Jesus to get to his now-dead daughter to bring her back to life? But Jesus didn't hurry. He didn't rush. He stopped and He cared for people. In the very next verse, it shows Jesus spoke life and encouragement to this humble woman, and *then* He made His way to Jairus' home and healed his daughter.

Looking back, I wonder why my pump site issue and the ten minutes it took to fix were such a big deal. The kids still got to summer camp just fine. Jesus faced situations of life and death and handled them with such grace, while what turned out to be a minor issue of my day threw my thought life spiraling.

So what's my point? Interruptions happen. Especially for people who deal with diabetes. That's just life. You know it, and I know it. How we respond to it is what matters. Go to the one who was remarkably interruptible to help you navigate the interruptions of life this side of heaven.

God, thank You for these accounts of Jesus' life. Thank You for the examples He has shown through the way He spoke and the way He lived. God, this disease I deal with day in and day out provides constant interruptions that take my immediate attention. Help me to have the patience I need, a calm demeanor like Jesus, and peace to handle interruptions with grace for myself and others. Amen.

Reading

Mark 5, Matthew 8

Reflection

What sort of interruptions do you often face? How do you handle them? Are there ways you could better handle interruptions? Take those thoughts to God today in prayer.

thoughts + prayers

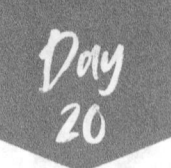

THE ILLUSION OF CONTROL

———————

I recently saw a coffee mug that said, "If you like roller coasters, I can't recommend diabetes enough." I had a good laugh and nodded my head in agreement. I had never considered that correlation before, but it seems true.

Like a roller coaster, diabetes can be unpredictable. It brings a unique set of twists and turns and ups and downs (highs and lows, literally). Just when you think you're coasting along with great blood sugar numbers, something changes and you're suddenly having repeat lows. And when you get that figured out, you either get sick and have insulin resistance or your doctor prescribes the "s word"…steroids. Hello, highs!

Even when we can point to what caused the change, we don't always understand why it caused it. There are too many variables that can affect blood sugar. It can sure be hard to pin down, and it can feel like you're out of control.

"Do you have good control?" People ask this question of people with diabetes, but isn't it funny? We want to control our diabetes, of course, to stay healthy and avoid complications and feel as good as we can. But is it possible for us to have control? I mean, really have control?

If you think about it, we mostly want to control our diabetes because we want to be in control of our lives. It's part of the human condition. We want things the way we prefer them.

We want to control all things. Even non-diabetes things. The guy who cuts us off in traffic. The weather—our outdoor plans cannot be ruined. The workday. The kids. How our spouse treats us. Our friendships. It's basically all of life.

But if we look deeper still, we see that our desire for control is the desire to be our own God. We want to call all the shots. We want to stop the storms from coming. We want to have control over our lives.

But we are not actually in control of anything—not our diabetes, and not much else. We live in a world of constant change, both around us and in us. And those things can change at warp speed.

When I recognize this, I'm glad I'm not in charge. I don't know all that God knows, and I can't see all that God sees. Life would be even more of a roller coaster if I were in full control.

> "For my thoughts are not your thoughts,
> neither are your ways my ways,"
> declares the Lord.
> "As the heavens are higher than the earth,
> so are my ways higher than your ways
> and my thoughts than your thoughts."
> Isaiah 55:8-9 (NIV)

God is immutable—He does not change. He knows all, sees all, and can do all. He is a master weaver of lives and stories and circumstances. That just blows my mind when I think about it. As Christ followers, we are not living our lives as though we are living our own story. We are each living a part of God's story as He works through us to reach this world for Him. He is in control.

Father, I thank You for Your goodness and faithfulness and trustworthiness today. There are times in this life that I want to be in full control. There are times I think I know best. And there are even times I feel like I can do it on my own. God, in those moments, I pray You would remind me of who You are—the unchanging, never failing, stable and secure God who is writing the story of my life. Help me rely on You and look to You in everything. Amen.

Reading

Numbers 23:19, Malachi 3:6, Hebrews 13:8, James 1:16-17

Reflection

Take time today to reflect and give thanks to God for writing the story of your life. Thank God that He is the one at the helm, that He is trustworthy, and that He is unchanging. We can take comfort in knowing that He is in control.

JESUS CHRIST IS THE SAME **YESTERDAY** AND **TODAY** AND **FOREVER.**

HEBREWS 13:8 (NIV)

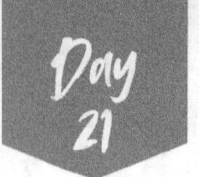

TRUE VALUE

I walked by the mirror the other day and caught a glimpse of my CGM peeking out from under my shirt sleeve. And I saw my insulin pump clipped at my waist making an awkward shape near the bottom of my shirt.

And what about the spot on my side where my insulin pump was yesterday? It's a bit red and looks slightly irritated. The place where my CGM was previously attached is a little bruised, and there's a black ring around where the tape used to be because I wore a dark sweatshirt one day and I guess some fuzz got stuck.

When I was taking multiple daily injections, I would have marks from the shots all over the outside of my thighs. And checking my blood sugar so often left dark little dots all over my fingertips.

There are times I feel like diabetes has a way of making me feel less attractive and less valuable. With bumps and bruises and equipment everywhere, how am I supposed to feel beautiful?

In a harsh and unforgiving world where beauty means being a certain size with a certain body shape and a certain hair style (and if you aren't, we'll just Photoshop you to appear that way), I'm positive I don't measure up to that standard. Not a chance.

But I have to stop myself. I need to take every thought, pair it up with God's Word, and find the ultimate truth about it all. I need to follow the instructions given to us in 2 Corinthians 10:5 to "take captive every thought to make it obedient to Christ."

When I do this, I am reminded that this world is not my home, and those who follow Christ cannot use this world's flawed benchmarks to define beauty. It doesn't match up. God created me in His image, and I am beautiful. Scars and all.

Being conscious of appearance is not a new thing. In the Old Testament, the people expected their leaders to look a certain way—they were to be tall, rugged, strapping men who look like they could easily win battles and slay lions at the same time. And Samuel thought so too. When he saw the first of Jesse's sons, based on his appearance alone, Samuel said, "Surely the Lord's anointed stands here before the Lord."

But God used this opportunity to share something insightful with Samuel. And we can apply it to our lives today.

> *Do not consider his appearance or his height, for I have rejected him. The Lord does not look at the things people look at. People look at the outward appearance, but the Lord looks at the heart.*
> 1 Samuel 16:7 (NIV)

And so God revealed David, the smallest and youngest brother, as Israel's future king.

You are God's creation, created in His image and with a purpose. Be reminded today that the condition of your heart is more valuable to God than the outward appearance this world values so much. Give your heart the focus it needs.

Are you allowing God to work in your heart through prayer and reading His Word? Are you giving and serving others in some capacity that will help set your heart right? Seek His guidance and allow Him to direct you in every part of life and align your heart with His.

Lord, thank You for the lesson You shared with Samuel. What a needed reminder for me. Thank You for teaching me what is more valuable to You. God, this world is drowning in things that oppose Your Word. I pray You would help me to see the difference plainly, to remember Your ways are best, and to trust Your guidance—even if everyone around me is rowing in the opposite direction. Amen.

Reading

Psalm 100, Psalm 139:14, Genesis 1:27

Reflection

Take a few moments and journal your thanks to God for seeing past what this world sees to what is more valuable inside. Pray for any help and healing your heart needs in this area.

_____

_____

_____

_____

_____

_____

_____

_____

_____

_____

_____

_____

thoughts + prayers

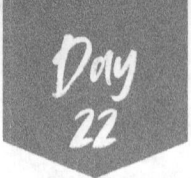

Day 22

OUR NEED FOR DEPENDENCE

When I was first diagnosed, I remember my family learning to count carbs and use a blood sugar meter. We all learned how to give insulin injections and treat lows. We went through various educational classes to learn to manage things independently before we left the hospital.

I vividly remember this petite lady with short, curly, reddish hair who taught us the nutrition side of things. She was a spitfire full of energy, and she talked a million miles a minute. We had to ask her to repeat herself quite often. But we learned. It was crucial that we understood the day-to-day things we needed to be successful.

Even at just 12 years old, I quickly started taking care of myself independently. I was testing my blood sugar multiple times a day and giving myself shots. I knew when I felt low, and I would drink juice to correct it.

There is a focus on independence in both diabetes and in our society in general. In our culture, we raise our children to be independent. That's a parent's role—to raise kids to be self-sufficient citizens. Independence all around us.

I was then (and still am now) an independent, type A personality most of the time. And it is good to know how to care for yourself—don't get me wrong. There is a need for that. But there's something we shouldn't forget. Something that is altogether too easy to overlook when we feel like we can do it all on our own.

We need to be dependent on the Lord.

The Psalmist wrote such a beautiful song of dependence that we need to just read the whole thing and soak in every single word.

> *I lift up my eyes to the mountains—*
> *where does my help come from?*
> *My help comes from the Lord,*
> *the Maker of heaven and earth.*
> *He will not let your foot slip—*
> *he who watches over you will not slumber;*
> *indeed, he who watches over Israel*
> *will neither slumber nor sleep.*
> *The Lord watches over you—*
> *the Lord is your shade at your right hand;*
> *the sun will not harm you by day,*
> *nor the moon by night.*
> *The Lord will keep you from all harm—*
> *he will watch over your life;*
> *the Lord will watch over your coming and going*
> *both now and forevermore.*
> *Psalm 121 (NIV)*

By day and by night, our loving Father watches over us. He is our keeper both now and forever more. He is our source of life, and without Him we can do nothing.

Without God, where would you be? Without His guidance and help, how would your life look different today?

It shouldn't take a blustery storm to knock us off our feet for us to realize our dependence on God. We need Him every day. We need to wake each morning and thank the Lord. We should pray for His presence and guidance daily. Our very dependence on God equips our independence.

God, thank You for these beautiful words in the book of Psalms. And thank You for the reminder of my dependence on You. You are my creator and sustainer. Even through the hard times and challenging circumstances in life, I know You are with me. Father, help me to push against the urge to want to do things on my own. Help me look to You and depend on You in every situation. Help me abide in You as my source of life, knowing I can do nothing apart from You. Amen.

Reading

John 15:1-8

Reflection

Read the additional verses in the book of John listed above and consider how a constant connection with God can help you understand your need for dependence on Him. Journal your thoughts or a prayer on the lines provided.

_____

_____

_____

_____

_____

_____

_____

_____

_____

_____

_____

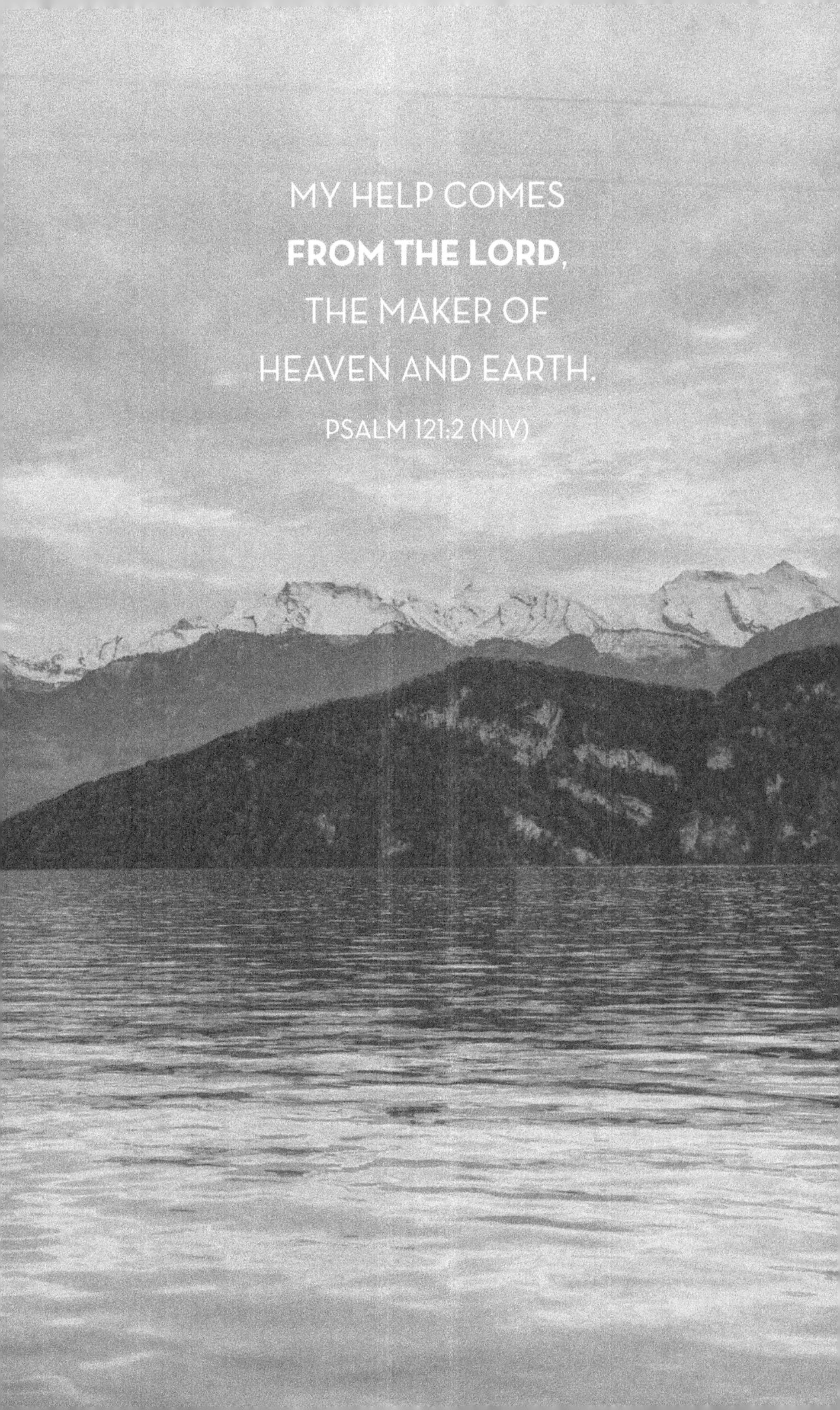

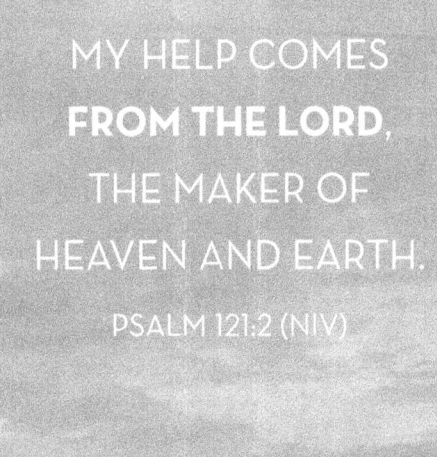

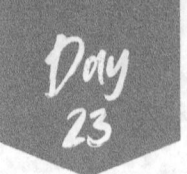

A NEW PRAYER

A few years ago, I discovered I really enjoyed prayer journaling. It wasn't much of a surprise—I have always enjoyed writing. But this gave me a creative outlet as well. And I had a habit of using that time specifically to pray for other people's prayer requests, which I also enjoyed.

While writing my prayers for other people, verses would come to mind for that particular person or their situation. I would share that with them with the hope of encouraging them. Sometimes those verses changed my perspective and even adjusted my prayers for them.

The thoughts that led me to write this devotional have shifted my prayers about diabetes specifically. As I mentioned in the introduction to this book, this isn't just about diabetes anymore. It's about how I can use the talents and gifts God has given me, along with the challenges of this disease, to point people to Him and give Him glory.

Today my prayers look more like this:

Help me abide in You.
I pray that I recognize God is with me as I battle this chronic illness day in and day out. I know He is my source of strength and peace and endurance. John 15:5 says, "I am the vine; you are the branches. Whoever abides in me and I in him, he it is that bears much fruit, for apart from Me you can do nothing" (ESV). Lord, help me abide.

Help me to be grateful for what I have.
Boy, has diabetes care come a long, long way in a relatively short time. It's easy to grumble when things aren't going right, but I should be thankful for what I have. I need to follow the words of the Apostle Paul. He said, "Rejoice always, pray continually, give thanks in all circumstances; for this

is God's will for you in Christ Jesus" (1 Thessalonians 5:16-18 NIV). Lord, help me to be thankful.

Help me to help others in Your name.
Jesus Himself, in the sermon on the mount, said, "Let your light shine before others, that they may see your good deeds and glorify your Father in heaven" (Matthew 5:16 NIV). How can I see having diabetes as an opportunity to help others and glorify God? I pray God will help me see those opportunities to glorify Him through all I do, ultimately pointing people to Him. Lord, help me to help others.

Help me to want You more than anything else.
While I do have the promise of no illness in heaven, I still live in this fallen and broken world. So as long as I'm here, am I worshiping this promise I'll have down the road, or am I worshiping the One who made it? It's easy for me to be hyper-focused on diabetes in the moment, but I pray God would help me want Him more than anything else. To be in a right relationship with God, I need to have a deep desire for the One who provides the healing more than I crave the cure itself. He is ultimately the creator and sustainer of life. "He is before all things, and in Him all things hold together" (Colossians 1:17 NIV). Lord, help me to desire You.

What are your prayers about diabetes? Do you pray for God to just stop the storm and take it all away? Do you only pray for a cure? While we wait for the long-term answers to those prayers, I encourage you to simply focus on God being with you and working through you. Allow Him to change your perspective. This life of ours is a blip on the radar in view of eternity. How can you allow God to help you use all the time you have for His glory?

> *Therefore, we do not lose heart. Though outwardly we are wasting away, yet inwardly we are being renewed day by day. For our light and momentary troubles are achieving for us an eternal glory that far outweighs them all. So we fix our eyes not on what is seen, but on what is unseen, since what is seen is temporary, but what is unseen is eternal.*
> *2 Corinthians 4:16-18 (NIV)*

God, thank You for prayer, and for wanting relationship with me. Thank You for the power of prayer and how You can work through any situation to bring about good. I pray today that You would refocus me with an eternal perspective. Help me to see ways I can bring You glory through this illness. Help me to help others while I abide in You as my strength and my sustainer. Amen.

Reading

Jeremiah 29:12-13, 1 John 5:14

Reflection

Today, consider how God can work through you to reach others for Him. How can He grow your faith through this experience? God can use diabetes for His glory so that our suffering through a chronic illness isn't for nothing. Pray that He would shape you, mold you, and refine you through it.

_____

_____

_____

_____

_____

_____

_____

_____

_____

thoughts + prayers

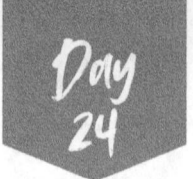

Day 24

GENEROUS GRACE

I had been on hold for about 12 minutes with some pretty fancy elevator music by the time the receptionist answered my call. I let her know I needed to schedule an appointment with my endocrinologist. It was unusual that I hadn't set one up at the end of my last appointment, but I was glad I realized it; I was due to see him in about six weeks. She looked at the schedule and offered me her first available appointment—five months away. I suppose a video visit would have to do in the meantime.

Later that morning, I returned a call to the pharmacy to confirm the refill of a prescription and asked when it would be ready to pick up. I decided I would go later that afternoon, after I finished working and getting the kids from school.

When I got home, I found a bill in the mail for the last 90 days of pump supplies from our mail order pharmacy. Another bill to pay. I filed it away to be taken care of later that week.

Really, none of this is abnormal for someone dealing with a chronic illness like diabetes. It's just extra work above and beyond what we would be required to do in the case that we didn't have diabetes to manage. This is simply the day in and day out stuff. The muck. The junk that must be done. The extra work it takes to stay on top of it. And it actually can be a whole lot of work.

I find myself working in other areas of my life as well. To keep up with the kids' school and activity schedules, to wash the never-ending pile of laundry, to cook and clean up the meals for the family…the list goes on.

I tend to be a pretty task-focused person, but if I'm not careful, all this work will bleed into my walk with God. I can start "working" to do all the right things…in reading, in worship, in prayer…even though I know nothing is based on my work.

The risk is in allowing the work—any type of work—to overtake my relationship with God. But thank God for His ocean full of grace that we don't have to work to earn His love. We are so very blessed that He has created us Himself and loves us always.

And thank God He chose to send His one and only Son as a spotless and blameless man, to stand in our place, to take the punishment for our sins, to rise again, and to defeat death and the grave. Through this beautiful and selfless sacrifice that we could never possibly work enough to earn, we can be reunited with God the Father. It's not because of our work, but it is offered to us as a gift.

> *For the wages of sin is death, but the free gift of God is eternal life in Christ Jesus our Lord.*
> *Romans 6:23 (ESV)*

Yes, dealing with diabetes is a lot of work. But even more important than managing this chronic illness is our salvation. Thank God for His ultimate rescue plan for us and that we can now be with Him in eternity when we place our trust and hope in Jesus.

It's not about the work we've done, but the work Jesus did on the cross on our behalf. Our God is extravagantly generous in offering us the free gift of life. And for that, we can be forever grateful.

> *For by grace you have been saved through faith. And this is not your own doing; it is the gift of God, not a result of works, so that no one may boast.*
> *Ephesians 2:8-9 (ESV)*

God, thank You for Your unending love that will never fail. Thank You for Your amazing and selfless plan to rescue us all through Your Son's sacrifice. You are so incredibly generous. God, when I feel the load of work to manage my diabetes, remind me that You love me. Remind me that my salvation is more important than the work of this world. And remind me that it's not something I can work to earn but a gift through Jesus. Help me to offer myself generous grace and be thankful each and every day for Jesus. Amen.

Reading

John 3:16, 2 Corinthians 5:21

Reflection

Choose one of the verses of additional reading listed above, and write it on the lines provided. Read it over and let it really sink in. What does this verse reveal to you about the character of God?

_____

_____

_____

_____

_____

_____

_____

_____

thoughts + prayers

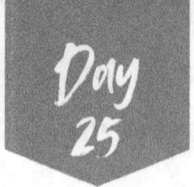

Day 25

FROM FEAR TO PRAYER

It was 10:30 that night. The house was dark. I had just snuggled into bed when I heard our daughter get up across the hall. I went to check on her and found her in the bathroom again. "Mom, it feels like I'm always using the bathroom anymore," she said. "And my throat is always dry, so I feel like I want to drink water all the time, too."

Time stood still for me—just long enough for one of my deeply-rooted fears to race ahead of my brain's capacity to function calmly.

I asked her to finish up in the bathroom and get a quick drink so we could check her blood sugar (which, of course, didn't exactly thrill her).

The relief I felt at the result on the meter allowed my heart rate to return to normal. Our daughter went to bed, and we were all sound asleep in no time. Interestingly, her symptoms were gone the next day.

But I found myself wondering later, what would it have been like had we been concerned about the results? What if she went on to continue having these classic type 1 symptoms? What if she ended up being diagnosed?

Have you ever worried about someone being diagnosed? I want so badly to trust that God would protect her. He protected her as I carried her before she was born. He created a completely healthy baby inside my chronically ill body—that's quite a miracle to me! So why wouldn't He protect her from this?

The trouble is, we live in this crazy world full of disease. Millions of people in this world have diabetes. What's to say my daughter will never be diagnosed? I can't prevent type 1, so what can I do?

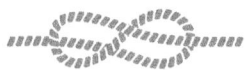

I pray. I pray that God would protect my daughter. I have prayed that prayer and will continue to do so. But something recently changed in my heart that shifted my prayer for her. I still pray for her protection, but I also pray that, if she is ever diagnosed, God will be with her through it. That God will be with me through it. That He will provide comfort and guidance through it all.

God is always with us through everything we face. We know that promise from multiple places in scripture.

> *Fear not, O Zion; let not your hands grow weak. The Lord your God is in your midst, a mighty one who will save.*
> *Zephaniah 3:16a-17a (ESV)*

Here we have one of God's many "fear not" phrases found so often in the Bible. Why? Because we are prone to fear, and God knows it's unnecessary. For the Lord our God is with us. He is in our midst.

Thank God today for His presence, and ask Him for guidance through the hard circumstances and fears you face. Let's also teach our children and others we influence not to fear, but to seek Him through it all. When He is with us, we need not fear.

Lord, what a privilege it is to live this life You have given me. Thank You for being ever-present in my life. Circumstances in this world can be challenging and painful, and sometimes my fears get out ahead of my reality. I pray You would help me rely on Your guidance and strength to get through. Remove my fears by reminding me of Your presence today. Amen.

Reading

Psalm 139:7-10; John 14:27

Reflection

What fears do you have? How do you process through those fears? What can you find in today's devotion and the verses listed above to comfort you and recenter your mind? Write your thoughts on the lines provided, and pray for God's help. Let Him wash away your fears and fill you with trust in Him.

YOUR RIGHT HAND WILL **HOLD ME** FAST.

PSALM 139:10 (NIV)

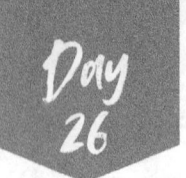

COMPRESSION

I woke to my CGM alert going off overnight because my number was reading low. I didn't feel low, so I checked my blood sugar manually and learned I wasn't actually low. My CGM was reading off, and I realized I had been laying on it while I was asleep. I'm typically very aware of where everything is when I sleep, and I'm able to avoid laying on the various things attached to my body, but evidently not this time.

This is called a "compression low," which is just a way of saying the sensor is being squashed and it's not able to get an accurate reading. Luckily, if it truly is a compression low and not an emergency, rolling over to relieve the pressure is about all it takes to fix it. But in the meantime, you have a CGM graph that looks like you're falling off a scary cliff. Oh... good ol' compressions lows. They're typically best at 3am. *(Ask me how I know.)*

What is intriguing though is how alike my CGM and I can be: when my CGM sensor is under pressure, it doesn't perform well. I usually don't function well when I am compressed either. When I'm feeling squeezed and pressured, I often buckle. And so did Peter at one crucial point in his life of following Jesus.

Go with me for a moment to Mark chapter 14. Peter, one of the first disciples and a super close friend to Jesus, had just been told at the last supper that he would deny Jesus three times before the rooster crowed. Peter declared in verse 31, "Even if I have to die with you, I will never disown you." He certainly believed in his own full allegiance to Christ.

But later, after Jesus was arrested, a servant of one of the high priests plotting to kill Jesus recognized Peter. When she confronted him as being as a follower of Jesus, he immediately denied it. That was once. Then he denied Christ twice more that night. Three times Peter folded under the

pressure. It was too much for him to bear. And when he realized what he had done, when he heard sound of the rooster's crow breaking through the crisp outdoor air, he remembered Jesus' words and broke down in tears.

Although he buckled under the pressure of this situation, he was later restored. John recorded Peter's restoration so beautifully in his gospel. In chapter 21, Jesus asks Peter in the presence of other disciples, "Do you love me?" three times. Peter pledged his love and devotion to Jesus each time, and he was restored. Peter went on to become a pillar of the Christian faith.

God ultimately wants restoration for all His children. He wants to use the pressure-filled experiences in our lives to help us, teach us, and heal us—as long as we will allow it.

What shows up when you are feeling compressed? Allow God to work in you during those times. He can act through the hardship to build and shape you to be more like Jesus. God's goal is that we are ultimately sanctified and transformed more and more into the likeness of His Son. Allow Him that space to work. Find Him and lean into Him in those times. Ask for His strength. Ask for His healing. Ask for His restoration.

> *And after you have suffered a little while, the God of all grace, who has called you to his eternal glory in Christ, will himself restore, confirm, strengthen, and establish you. To him be the dominion forever and ever. Amen.*
> 1 Peter 5:10 (ESV)

Lord, thank You for this beautiful picture of restoration. Thank You for the impact Peter had on so many lives during his ministry, and that he still reaches so many today through Your Word. Today, Lord, I pray for myself in the times that I feel the pressure mounting in my life, for those days that I feel squeezed and pulled and crushed. Those can be such hard days to maintain my composure and show the fruit of the spirit to others. But I pray You would help me to do just that. Guide and direct my thoughts and actions in those times. Work in my mind and heart to use those instances to mold and shape me to look more and more like Jesus. Amen.

Reading

Mark 14:66-72, John 21:15-19

Reflection

How do you respond to pressure? What do you do when you sense it mounting? Consider these questions and write a prayer below for God to help you respond well using His strength. Ask God to help you grow through these circumstances and pray that you would be open to follow His leading.

_____

_____

_____

_____

_____

_____

thoughts + prayers

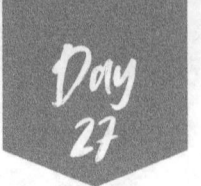

Day 27

BUILDING TRUST

"I just need some time to build trust before I would try anything like that again." That was my answer to the rep training me to use my new insulin pump when she asked if I was interested in using a closed-loop system in the future.

In case you are unfamiliar with closed-loop technology, it's a system in which you wear both a continuous glucose monitor and an insulin pump at the same time. Then you set them up to "talk" to each other and adjust doses to prevent lows and highs on their own. It's as close to an external pancreas as someone with diabetes can currently get. It sounds kind of like a dream, doesn't it?

But a few years ago, I gave this whole closed-loop thing a whirl, and it crashed and burned in nothing short of disaster. My diabetes was actually harder to control because the CGM I wore wasn't reading my blood sugars accurately, so my pump was dosing based off of inaccurate data. I lost countless hours of sleep, on top of losing sleep from having a five-month-old baby at the time. It was affecting my mood, my parenting, my marriage, and maybe even my sanity. My otherwise-well-controlled diabetes was suddenly a nightmare. And the alerts would not stop beeping, remind me of the struggle at all hours of the day and night.

In the case this system is working well for you, that's wonderful! But I have found over the years that we all need to make individual treatment choices, and that's ok. It's hard for me to put my trust in something that I know from experience can fail me. Thankfully, the rep understood and encouraged me to take the time I need to build trust.

While I may never trust a closed-loop system enough to try it again, I do trust God. He will never fail me. He is always faithful.

> *For the word of the LORD is right and true;*
> *he is faithful in all he does.*
> Psalm 33:4 (NIV)

God has shown Himself to be faithful and trustworthy throughout the Bible. He doesn't promise we won't face hardship, but He promises to be there with us through it. Even in the struggle, He is there. He is always present. He will never fail.

Where do you place your trust? I mean your deep-down ultimate trust. It's honestly pretty easy to place trust in other things like friends, career, financial status, and health. But those things give us a false sense of security. Friends can betray us, careers can end, finances can become unstable, and health can deteriorate. Everything in this world around us can fail. But God will not fail.

> *Some trust in chariots and some in horses, but we trust in the*
> *name of the LORD our God.*
> Psalm 20:7 (NIV)

God, You are such a good Father in that You are faithful every single day. Thank You that I can trust in You knowing You will never fail me. The things of this world can come calling for my attention and allegiance. But, God, I pray You would help me be faithful in return to You. Help me not to place my trust in other things that will fail me, but always only in You. Amen.

Reading

Proverbs 3:5, Isaiah 41:10, 2 Timothy 2:13

Reflection

Take a moment and consider where you place your trust. What in this world continues to call your name and beg for your attention and allegiance? How can you shift your perspective to trusting God through it all? Make some notes and pray today about being fully anchored and fully trusting in the name of the Lord our God.

THINGS I PLACE MY TRUST IN:

_____

_____

_____

_____

HOW I CAN SHIFT TO TRUST GOD:

_____

_____

_____

_____

IF WE ARE FAITHLESS,
HE **REMAINS** FAITHFUL.

2 TIMOTHY 2:13 (NIV)

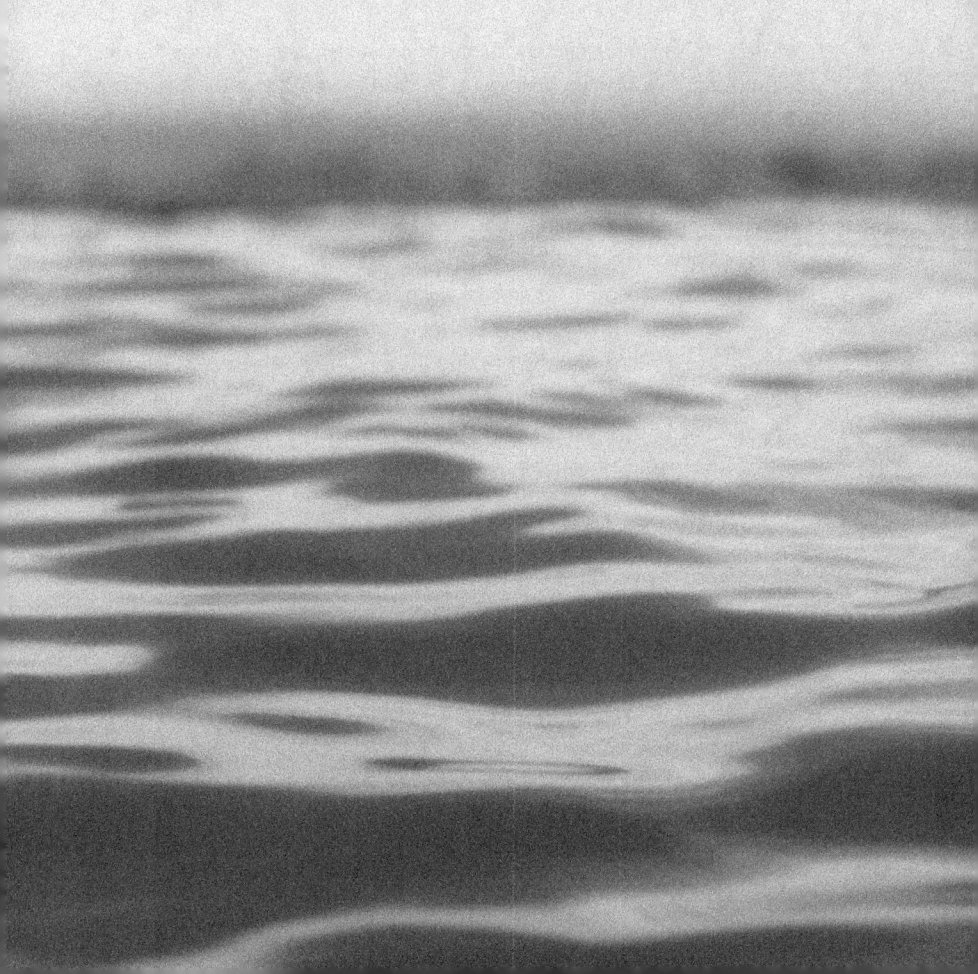

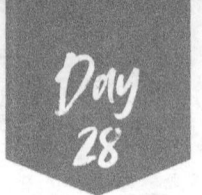
Day 28

PERFECT PEACE

Insulin? Check.
Pump site changes? Check.
Alcohol wipes? Check.
Glucose gummies? Check.
Juice boxes? Check.
Extra CGM sensors? Check.
Emergency supplies? Check.

I can feel the anxiety creep up my throat as I pack my bags for the weekend trip. I charge my meter just in case I need it as a backup to my CGM. Do I have enough testing strips? I'd better check.

Preparing to leave the comfort of my home, where I know I have all I need at hand, causes my mind and heart to race. The "what if" scenarios fly high—the scenarios that have never actually happened in real life at home, but I'm somehow convinced will happen while I'm away.

I finally get to a point with my packing list that I realize what's going on. I close my eyes. I take a deep breath. I remind myself that I have all I need. I've packed all I can. I will survive with all the supplies I have (the supplies I have set out and double checked already).

While it's important to take a moment to pack all I need, I can't dwell and allow it to make me anxious with worry.

Now, I need to calm my racing mind with reassurance and truth.

When my thoughts are going off the rails with anxiety and worry about something in my life, something as "simple" as packing for a trip, my mind is not on God. My mind is on worries of what may come, what may happen. Not real things, you understand.

But the prophet Isaiah reassures me:

> You keep him in perfect peace
> whose mind is **stayed** on you,
> because he **trusts** in you.
> Isaiah 26:3 (ESV)

I will fully admit I'm a grammar junkie, but I really love the way this verse is worded.

This isn't just an occasional thought going God's way, but stayed, meaning fixed. As in not going anywhere. An immovable focus on God. Our minds are generally stayed on whatever we trust. My mind can be stayed on God because of my trust in Him. And I know I can continually trust in Him.

Only when I place my trust in and focus my mind on God, can God keep me in perfect peace. When I am aligned with Him and focused on Him fully, trusting Him in all areas of my life, is when the raging seas in my mind calm and I can experience His gift of peace.

> Let the peace of Christ rule in your hearts, since as members of one body you were called to peace. And be thankful.
> Colossians 3:15 (NIV)

Lord, thank You for the beautiful words from Your prophet Isaiah. Thank You for the peace only You can provide. God, there are so many situations in life with diabetes that can divert my attention, shift my thoughts, and encourage my mind to wander from You. I pray today for Your refreshment. Renew my mind and fix my eyes on You. Amen.

Reading

Matthew 6:25-34, Philippians 4:6-7

Reflection

What is your mind stayed on? Where do you place your trust? Do you experience the perfect peace that can only come from God? Take time as you go about your day today to inventory what you focus your mind on. Go to God this evening with what you learn. Praise Him for being your focus, or ask for His help in renewing your mind and setting your gaze on Him.

thoughts + prayers

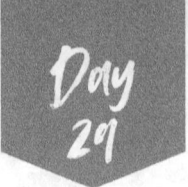

DIABETES IS TEMPORARY

———————

Shortly after we got married, Nick and I started playing tennis at nearby courts. It was a fun way to spend the weekend, get in some exercise, and gloat a little when you won. But it wasn't long until swinging the racket sent a sharp pain through my right shoulder. A few weeks later, I couldn't reach across my body to buckle my seat belt to drive. Then I wasn't able to get clothes down off the shelf in my closet. My arm simply wouldn't move that way anymore.

After a short period of blissfully wishing it would all just go away, I faced reality and asked my doctor what he thought was going on. He posed a few questions, measured my range of motion, and said very frankly, "You have a frozen shoulder."

He went on to tell me there was basically inflammation in the joint preventing full range of motion, and that physical therapy should help. But I didn't understand. This was the first I had ever even heard of a frozen shoulder, and I wanted to know why this was happening. His answer? "We don't fully know of a specific cause for this issue, but we do know it is common in people with diabetes."

Have you had a conversation like this? Sitting across from a doctor to learn how diabetes has caused some form of physical complication is hard. It's hard to hear. It's hard to understand. And yet, there are countless ways for various parts of our bodies to fail somehow due to diabetes.

We live in a world overflowing with brokenness and disease, chronic illness and pain. The difference-maker for me, and for all my brothers and sisters in Christ, is that my hope isn't in this fallen and broken world. Because I believe in Jesus and trust in Him, God promises that one day in heaven I will have a new body that isn't broken or diseased, chronically ill, or full of pain.

2 Corinthians 5:2 captures this idea so well, especially in the New Living Translation: "We grow weary in our present bodies, and we long to put on our heavenly bodies like new clothing."

What about you? Do you ever grow weary? Do you feel that longing? Do you yearn for the day you will be made new? It will be nothing short of a beautiful and glorious miracle to experience this renewed body in heaven in the overwhelming presence of *Jehovah Rapha*, the God who heals. One day He will make me new. Fully new. Through this eternal lens, I can say it with certainty: diabetes is temporary.

> *He will wipe every tear from their eyes, and there will be no more death or sorrow or crying or pain. All these things are gone forever.*
> Revelation 21:4 (NLT)

Heavenly Father, thank You for Your Word that gives me such hope in Jesus, heaven, and the ultimate restoration of my body. I pray You would remind me that You are faithful and that Your promises are true. Through the hard conversations, the days of pain and illness, and the failing of my body, refresh my mind. Help me to remember this earth and this earthly body are not my home. Remind me daily of Your amazing promise of healing. Amen.

Reading

2 Corinthians 5:1-10, Revelation 21:1-7, Philippians 3:21

Reflection

What does diabetes look like for you on a daily basis? How does God's promise of a renewed body transform your daily journey with diabetes? Take time to read through the additional readings above and consider this eternal hope. Spend a moment in thought and prayer today to renew your faith in Jesus as you reflect on this eternal perspective. Thank God for His ultimate healing and the hope we have in heaven.

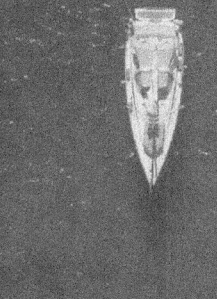

FOR WE
LIVE BY FAITH,
NOT BY SIGHT.
2 CORINTHIANS 5:7 (NIV)

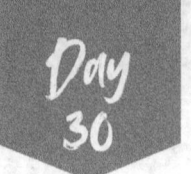

DROP ANCHOR

In the fall of 2022, southwest Florida was pummeled by Hurricane Ian. Ranked as a Category 4 storm at landfall, it wreaked havoc to say the least. Having family there, I was glued to the live stream of their local news station while they braced as best they could for its arrival.

I listened as the news crew gave updates on the storm's path. I watched as they showed footage of water flooding the streets and buildings near the shore. I saw images of boats piled on top of each other, trees uprooted, and beaches destroyed. It's not surprising to know it was the deadliest hurricane to hit the state of Florida since 1935.*

What does this have to do with diabetes? While locals were dealing with power outages for days on end due to the storm, people using rechargeable insulin pumps were praying for electricity to power their devices. Those with supply orders shipping to their homes were hoping the delivery vehicles could make it through the streets before they ran out of the medical supplies they needed. It was difficult to get to a grocery store or pharmacy for anything, and it was even harder to find the gas to get there.

In a crisis—and really always—we followers of Jesus need to make sure we are anchored in Him. Storms will come. Wild winds will blow. Floods will rise. And it doesn't have to be related to diabetes. Things in any part of our lives can take us off guard. All kinds of happenings in life will try to lift our anchor and carry us away from Jesus.

Some happenings are big, like Hurricane Ian. And some start small. We get "too busy" for God. We prioritize something else in a season of life. Or we simply lose focus for a while. We may not even realize it's happening at first. But little by little, we drift away. Not until we look back do we realize how far we've gone.

My point is this: drop anchor now. Don't wait for the storm. Anchor yourself in Jesus today. Truly, strongly, deeply anchor. And do it again every day. He is our source of life and our hope in times of trouble. Being anchored in Jesus is something we must do continually and intentionally. That's the only way we can be sure that the storms of life don't blow us off course when they come.

May we all continually anchor our souls in Jesus every day of our lives.

> We have this hope as an anchor for the soul, firm and secure.
> Hebrews 6:19 (NIV)

God, You are not blown by the winds and tossed by the waves. You are our steadfast Heavenly Father. Thank You for Your stability and security. I can begin to drift away from time to time, Lord, when the pressures of this world close in. I pray today You would help me remain in You. Hold me fast and help me to be anchored well each and every day. Amen.

Reading

Psalm 46:1-3, Psalm 62:1-2, Isaiah 26:3

Reflection

Now that we are drawing to a close together, how will you continue to be anchored in Jesus? How will you faithfully dive into God's Word tomorrow? How will you remain in prayer? How will you surround yourself with community that will hold you accountable? Who can you reach out to when you need help? Use the following pages to make notes, write down your ideas, and pray for God's guidance as you prayerfully consider these questions.

---

*https://en.wikipedia.org/wiki/Hurricane_Ian

MIGHTIER THAN THE THUNDERS OF MANY WATERS, MIGHTIER THAN THE WAVES OF THE SEA, **THE LORD ON HIGH** IS MIGHTY!

PSALM 93:4 (ESV)

GRATITUDE

This book would not exist without the following people.

I owe endless gratitude to Nick—my husband, pastor, and late-night theology checker. Thank you for asking hard questions and keeping me in line, and for giving me the margin to do this work. xo.

To my parents who are always behind me with their support...thank you for being real with me in conversations about diabetes. Thank you for being strong in the face of my diagnosis, although I can only imagine how difficult it was. You are both so courageous.

Brandy, you are my encourager friend I couldn't do without. We can talk about diabetes and relate to each other all day long. But more importantly, we point each other to Jesus. Thank you for being my iron that sharpens iron.

Annette, my dear long-time designer friend...you are skilled beyond belief, and this book is beautiful because of you. I am honored to showcase your work around my words. THNK U from the bottom of my heart.

Ami, you make my thoughts and words flow so well. Thank you for your time, effort, prayer, and encouragement in editing this book. You're already hired for the next one, my friend.

And to Jesus. I have been blessed to view my chronic illness through the lens of the Bible. Thank You for showing me this perspective. And thank You for using something hard and challenging for good. Yet again. Please keep revealing Your truths and opening my eyes.

DID YOU ENJOY THIS BOOK?

Thank you for reading *Devotions on Diabetes: A 30-Day Journey to Anchor Your Soul*. Would you consider sharing this with someone? Here are a few ideas:

- Write a review where you purchased this book.

- Post about it on social media using #DevotionsOnDiabetes.

- Purchase a copy for a friend or family member.

- Sign up for weekly blog emails at DevotionsOnDiabetes.com.

- Connect with us online:
  Blog website: DevotionsOnDiabetes.com
  Facebook: Devotions On Diabetes
  Instagram: @DevotionsOnDiabetes

Thank you in advance!

www.ingramcontent.com/pod-product-compliance
Lightning Source LLC
Chambersburg PA
CBHW070430010526
44118CB00014B/1987